Dementia ~~Caregiver~~ Care Partner Guide

Expanded and Revised

Dementia ~~Caregiver~~ Care Partner Guide

Expanded and Revised

Practical Tips for Transforming
the Possibilities of Care

Teepa Snow, MS, OTR/L, FAOTA

Founder of Positive Approach to Care®

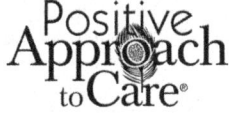

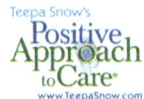

Efland, NC

This book was originally published by Cedar Village Retirement Community in Mason, OH, sponsored by The Schriber Family Foundation in memory of Louis and Isabel Schriber.

Neither Positive Approach nor any of its officers, directors, employees, or other representatives will be liable for any damages, special or consequential, or otherwise, arising out of or in connection with the use of this work, or any information contained therein.

Copyright © 2025 by Teepa Snow and Positive Approach, LLC
Edition #3
First Edition 2012

All rights reserved. No part of this book may be reproduced or transmitted in any form or by any means, electronic or mechanical, including photocopying, recording, or any information storage and retrieval system, without permission in writing from the author.

ISBN: 979-8-9859120-6-7 - Paperback
eISBN: 979-8-9859120-7-4 - eBook

Library of Congress Control Number: 2025902965

∞ This paper meets the requirements of ANSI/NISO Z39.48-1992 (Permanence of Paper)

Positive Approach, Positive Approach to Care, GEMS, and Hand-under-Hand are registered trademarks of Positive Approach, LLC, registered in the United States. Snow Approach, PAC, Positive Physical Approach, and PPA are trademarks of Positive Approach, LLC.

021925

Understanding the GEMS States of Brain Change and Learning to Shift from Caregiver to Care Partner

Discovering what's unique, remarkable, and even precious in the progression of dementia.

Helping you let go of what is missing and learn to celebrate and use what remains, making life worth living until the end of the journey.

A special thank you to Debi Newsom for her contributions to the original *Dementia Caregiver Guide* and for inspiring this revised edition.

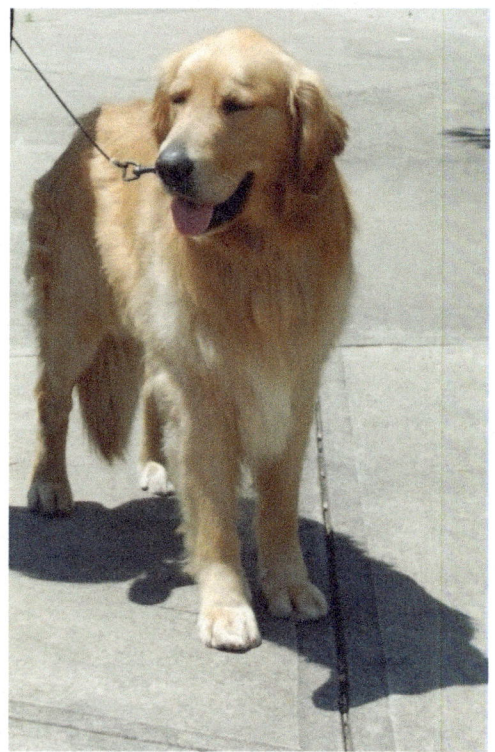

Debi's beloved and loyal golden retriever service dog, Gates.

"We must not see any person as an abstraction. Instead, we must see in every person a universe with its own secrets, with its own treasures, with its own sources of anguish, and with some measure of triumph."
—Elie Wiesel

Contents

How to Use This Guidebook — xiii
Key Aspects of the GEMS® States — xvii

GEMS® States Characteristics — 1
    Sapphire State — 1
    Diamond State — 4
    Emerald State — 10
    Amber State — 21
    Ruby State — 26
    Pearl State — 32
GEMS® State Support to Consider — 37
Hand-under-Hand® Support — 45
Positive Physical Approach™ (PPA™) — 55
Positive Personal Connectors (PPC) — 59
Positive Action Starters (PAS) — 61
Approaching an Individual Who Is Distressed — 63

Other Resources — 67
Conclusion — 77

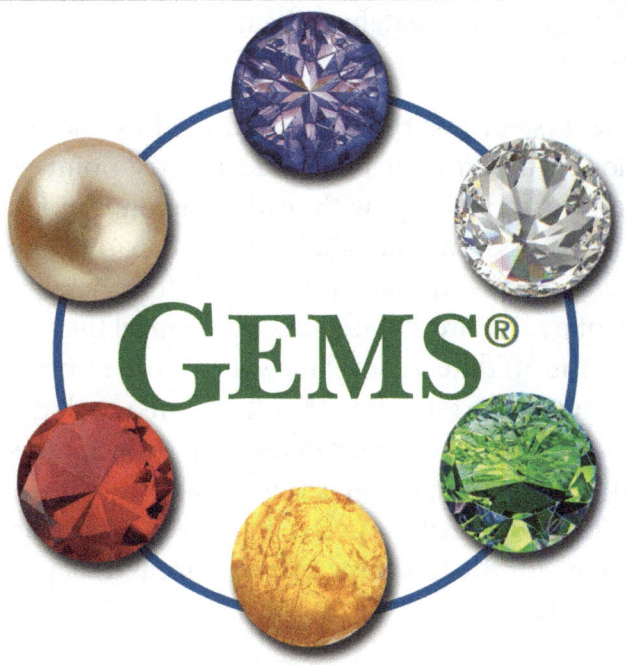

How to Use This Guidebook

This book is designed for those who support someone living with a changing brain. Its goal is to improve awareness of the shifts in brain states that occur due to dementia or other impairments in thinking, reasoning, or processing information.

With this understanding, we can provide better support and care, and help others live fully in their moment. When we appreciate what is changing and what is still possible, we can have interactions that are more positive, communication that is more productive, and care that is more effective and less challenging for all concerned.

Why Did I Develop the GEMS® States of Brain Change?

After working as an Occupational Therapist with existing dementia progression rating systems for more than twenty years, I found that while they each had elements I could use, they didn't quite adequately and empathetically show me the whole person.

One rating system was promoted and used by the Alzheimer's Assocation at the time. It contained a three-point scale, one to three, corresponding with early, middle, and late-stage dementia. This system does allow us to get an idea about where someone is in the disease process. Unfortunately, the vast majority of people are still not diagnosed until they are already well into the middle stage. Since it is new information for families and supporters, they are often thinking that dementia is still in an early stage. This can result in expectations that are too high for how the person is functioning at that time. What they don't realize is that they often have been experiencing early brain change for the last three to five years and may already be in a middle stage.

A second system, developed by Dr. Reisberg, is known as the Global Deterioration Scale (GDS). It is a seven-point scale, with one being no cognitive decline and seven being very severe cognitive decline (severe dementia). The emphasis is on what is being lost; what the person is no longer able to do and what performance abilities will deteriorate during that phase. It emphasizes that the pattern of loss most frequently mimics the opposite of normal growth and development we see in infants, children, and adolescents.

This system is fairly accurate if the person has a more typical dementia progression pattern, such as that seen in Alzheimer Disease. However, it can be less accurate for other types of dementia with uneven progression patterns, including Vascular, Lewy Body, and Frontotemporal dementias.

A third system was developed by an Occupational Therapist during her clinical work with people experiencing a variety of cognitive issues. The system is based on her Cognitive Disability Theory and the levels are called Allen Cognitive Levels. There are six levels, six being no cognitive impairment, and one being severely impaired. The strength of this system is that it focuses on more than just loss. It emphasizes the abilities and interests of individuals at each of the levels, and the environmental support and care behaviors that may be helpful. With this system, individuals may have a combination of levels present at one time and can move between levels throughout a day or task, depending on stressors and supports.

Although I liked and used this system, I felt it had a significant issue. The numbering is in the opposite direction compared to the other two systems, meaning we would always be having disagreements in rating simply because of our association of numbers. Also, numbers always have meaning: one is less than six, and first is better than sixth. Unfortunately, numbers generally indicate some sort of value statement: better than, less than, more than. In my view, people are not numbers, and their value does not change with changing brain abilities. They are simply different in those moments than at other times.

I wanted to create a system that could:

1. Help us see what remains and learn how to support and use those skills.

2. Provide consistent ways in which we can modify or structure the environment, the tasks, and our support for the best chance of success for each person in our care, based on what they can do and what they need help to do.

3. Allow us to talk with each other in a way that does not carry so much negativity and stigma.

4. Be used by lay people as well as professionals.

5. Talk about abilities in a way that is not hurtful or offensive to those who are living with brain change.

6. Look at ourselves, those of us with healthy or neurotypical brains, and our continually fluctuating abilities and brain states, so that we may be able to recognize our own status at a moment in time.

The GEMS® States system is my effort to simplify a very complex process into a structured approach for all involved, so that we may better care for and support those living with changing abilities, as well as ourselves.

Although I initially developed the GEMS States with the idea that they apply only to those living with dementia or another form of brain change, further refinement of the model helped me to realize that these brain states apply to all individuals in all phases of life. Even those with healthy brains will experience all GEMS States throughout the course of a typical day. For example, we will experience a Pearl State when we are sleeping or meditating, or an Amber State when we get completely caught up in an interesting experience and lose track of time and the bigger picture.

However, when someone is living with dementia, the structural changes in the brain significantly reduce their ability to shift quickly between states or sustain a brain state for any length of time. They will typically spend most of their time in a state that is not the Sapphire State.

Different forms of dementia will often result in different patterns of GEMS State shifts. For instance, with Vascular Dementia, abilities are quite variable, so someone may be in a Diamond State most of one day, and the next day they may spend the majority of their time in an Amber State. Awareness of an individual's GEMS State at any given moment of time, and being able to offer the support that is helpful for that particular GEMS State, is essential to effective care.

—Teepa

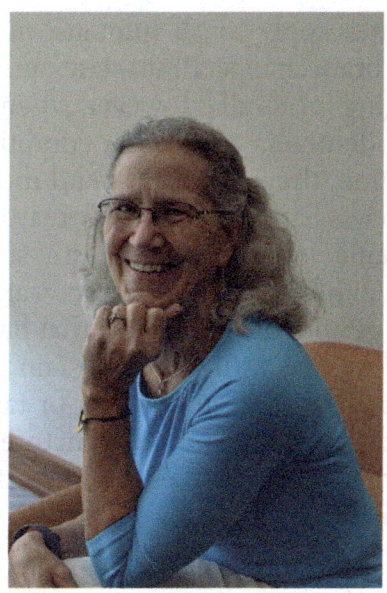

Teepa Snow, MS, OTR/L, FAOTA

Key Aspects of the GEMS® States

Why GEMS? I am committed to finding a more inclusive and positive way of seeing the brain changes that are associated with dementia, as well as our own brain plasticity and potential for change. I also am interested in using an inclusive range of brain state possibilities, rather than a more traditional labeling system that separates *us* from *them*. To me, all gemstones are beautiful and interesting. Each is unique. Each has noticeable characteristics that can be seen and identified. I also believe that in the right setting and with the right care, each gemstone can shine. For those living with dementia, we can provide support and care that promotes optimal abilities. We can acknowledge shifts that happen so that we can provide the right support in the moment. For care partners, recognizing our changing GEMS States throughout the day can help us put challenges in perspective and perhaps help us seek the support we need to keep us well throughout this journey of discovery! Five key points to remember about the GEMS States of Brain Change:

1. GEMS States apply to all humans, not just those living with brain change. Brain states and abilities are ever-changing for us all. However, when someone is living with dementia or another condition affecting brain function, they typically spend more time in a state that is not Sapphire, and they may well become more extreme in their shifts from state to state. They may either give little or no warning or not shift at all, despite using support that has previously worked. They may struggle to sustain a brain state for the duration of an interaction or task. This can be due to the changes in brain structure and wiring, or the environment or support mismatch they are experiencing.

2. Be aware of your own current GEMS State at any given moment, as this will impact your ability to effectively respond and support. Even if you have full cognitive abilities and typically function in a Sapphire State, factors such as surprises, unfamiliar environments, illness, circadian rhythms, sleep, and stress affect your brain state and cause it to shift.

3. GEMS States can and do vary during the course of each day. As we face different settings, tasks, and people, our ability to cope and respond may change regularly or unexpectedly. The existence and impact of other medical, emotional, and sensory conditions (vision, hearing, touch, balance, pain) can also affect GEMS States. Most of us, whether or not we are living with brain change, perform better when we are rested, focused, and alert than we do when we are tired, stressed, distracted, or in pain. Use what you see, hear, and experience to help determine where someone else is functioning at that moment. Then, adjust your expectations, support, and behavior to match what is happening for them. Possibly consider taking a short break, if you notice that your GEMS State is not a good match for your partner.

4. Individuals may show signs of different GEMS States at the same time. It turns out that different lobes and functions of the brain may be impacted in different ways at any moment in time. Your support may need to shift to better match the type of activity, sensory system, or most impacted area of function. If you are assisting someone and you are noticing this, choose the support that seems to match the majority of the indicators as a first try. Notice how it is working and modify as needed.

5. If there is a sudden or unexpected change in the GEMS State of an individual you are supporting, communicate this noticed change to all those who are monitoring the health and well-being of the person. The change may possibly indicate environmental or emotional distress, a physical problem, a health issue, or a condition that should be more carefully evaluated.

GEMS States are not negative labels. They are brain change indicators to help us better understand ourselves and those we support. When we experience a GEMS State shift, an effective friend, partner, or coworker will automatically move into a supportive mode and help us out, rather than becoming frustrated or accusing us of being stubborn, stupid, not paying attention, or not trying hard enough.

On the next page, there is a table with basic information on each of the GEMS States: the name of the state, characteristics of the state, and general behavioral features of an individual in that state. Both remaining abilities and key missing pieces are noted.

The following pages after the chart will explore the GEMS States in detail. Each GEMS State will be described, with remaining abilities highlighted and lost skills noted, and cues provided for offering optimal support for an individual in that state.

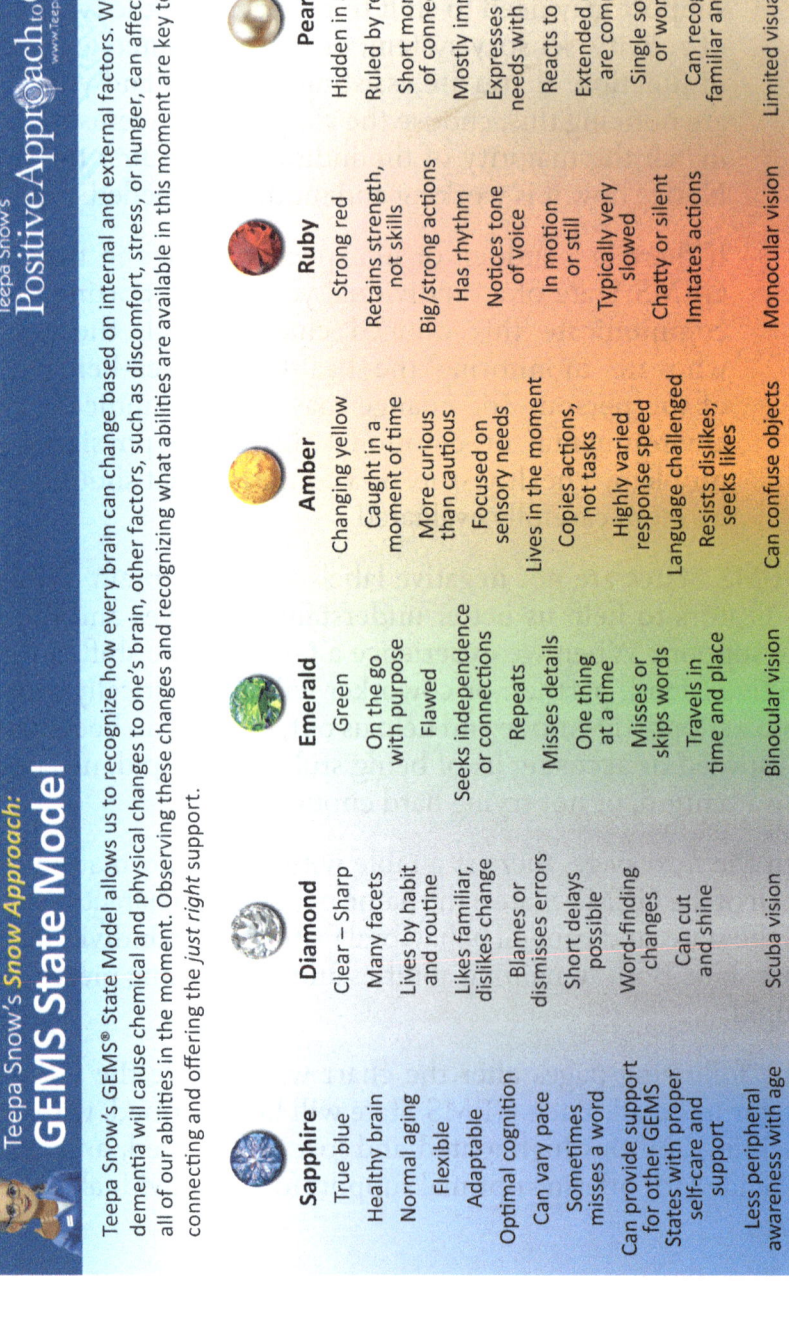

Dementia Care Partner Guide

What can I show/say/do to support a person in a particular GEMS State?

Based on what you observe, choose your response from the skills below to offer support.

My Skills	Sapphire	Diamond	Emerald	Amber	Ruby	Pearl
Responding to Their Vision	Greet, stay in visual field when interacting, use supportive stance (body to the side, face toward person)	Get visual attention, respect space/distance preferences, use directional signs and labels	Offer familiar gestures, use supportive stance, limit complex cues, present items for use in their center field of vision only	Show items, then gesture use. Point to direct attention. Eliminate items that could cause harm, but offer substitutions	Offer greeting matching speed, allow time to visually explore objects and you. One item/cue at a time. Exaggerate	Seek gaze by placing face in central field. Place objects within arm's length, first use gestures to show actions
Responding to Their Language	Ask permission to reduce background noise or change locations. Summarize or ask questions to confirm	Connect before sharing info. Acknowledge preferences and emotions. Empathize – Confirm their emotional state and then say I'm Sorry	Use preferred name, reflect key message they gave. Keep answers short/concrete. Pair words with gesture or object. Slow down, use pauses, instruct one step at a time	Use familiar greeting or name, smile or reflect their expression to acknowledge. Use only 2 or 3 words at a time. Pair words with gesture or object. Reinforce efforts (Good!; Keep going)	Use facial expression with greeting. Pair single word with gesture or object. Use song, counting, or rhythm to initiate or transition. Use vocal rhythm to change pace	Deepen your speech, slow your speech, use sounds (Ooh! Ummm) or single words (Good. Drink?), then combine motions with your words
Touching a Person	Shake hands, respect personal space preferences, get permission to touch	Shake hands, respect personal space preferences, get permission to touch. If showing distress – comforting hug or touch, only with permission	Use handshake greeting to note touch tolerance, use Hand-under-Hand (HuH) clasp when helping in intimate space, offer objects held the direction the person would hold/use them	Get visual and verbal permission, then touch at the hand first. To get started, use HuH to guide and direct. Offer substitutions – do not just take something away	Offer hand, wait for regard, move into HuH when greeting, place other hand on shoulder or joint when assisting. Use HuH for support, tasks, guiding	To reduce distress, move one hand at a time; other hand connect with shoulder or joint. For all care; slow, flat, solid touch. Extending limbs may cause harm
Getting a Person to Move/Do Something	Seek partnership. Ask for their support/help. Acknowledge pain or discomfort before acting	Appreciate their skill or background. Ask for their help, allow time, and offer options to watch, supervise, or do	Consider staying at edge of public space and gesturing with energy your desire for them to get up and join you, bring a prop to see	Demo what to do at arm's length in central visual field, then offer the object or use HuH to begin. Use gestures to signal getting up, after rising yourself	Say their name, do what you want them to do, then use single words only. Guide movement to help them begin, re-cue if needed	Greet, pause. Use counting or emphasis to help the person to know what is going to happen. Go SLOW, pause, watch for discomfort

*Hand-under-Hand Techniques

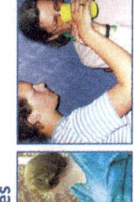
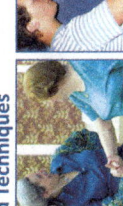
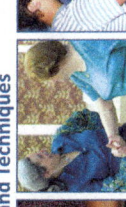
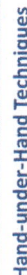

Hand-under-Hand® Positive physical Approach™

Learn more about Hand-under-Hand and other supporting techniques with videos and resources at **www.TeepaSnow.com**.

Copyright © 2006 - 2023 Positive Approach, LLC and Teepa Snow.
May not be duplicated or re-used without prior permission. V112023

Key Aspects of the GEMS® States

GEMS® States Characteristics

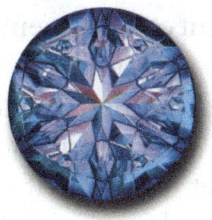

Sapphire State

Typical Aging

My brain is functioning and aging in a healthy manner. There may be some changes, but they tend to happen to everyone and have been gradually occurring over time since my late twenties. I am generally as I have always been. I cycle through all the GEMS States throughout the course of a day, but I am typically able to function in a Sapphire State when needed.

I am usually able to be flexible and adaptable, and I can consider the perspectives and points of view of others. I can still learn new things and change habits, but if I am an older individual, it may take longer and more effort on my part. Other health problems, sensory changes (vision problems, hearing changes, balance or coordination concerns), psychological or mental health concerns (depression, anxiety, personality disorders, etc.), medication effects or side effects, or chronic pain issues may affect my abilities and behavior, but generally, my cognitive function is stable.

Sometimes it may be hard for me to find a particular word, but I eventually get it, or at least am able to describe it well enough so that someone else can understand me. Word finding is harder if I am tired, ill, hurting, stressed, or trying to do too many things at one time. I may think out loud as I am doing things or working things through, giving myself cues and prompts—this is typical aging for a healthy, busy adult.

I can remember important commitments and information, even though I may need to use reminders, schedules, or lists. I will typically need to use aids for details and complex instructions or information. I may need repetition to learn complicated information and may get frustrated if you try to go too fast or point out that I am not as sharp as you expect me to be.

Honoring my preferences and choices whenever possible will result in improved interactions. If there is something you really want or need me to do, please first consider who I am and how I like to receive information, process details, and make decisions.

Note: If someone is not experiencing cognitive decline and has never had the flexibility or adaptability of those in a Sapphire State, the Diamond State may be their natural tendency. Try using the Diamond State tips in interactions and see if it might help.

Helpful Tips for Supporting Someone in a Sapphire GEMS State:

1. I will usually want time to make choices or decisions. Please offer the information and then let me think about it or listen to me talk about it before you need an answer.

2. I will typically resent a takeover unless I ask or want you to do so, or I may be comfortable with your choice if my goal is to spend time with you regardless of activity.

3. I can typically use logic and reason, so make use of what you know about me to help determine how, when, who, and what types of questions to ask, information to share, and support to offer, to get to a conclusion or decision.

4. If I have preferred learning styles or memory prompts, respect and honor my preferences. Specific examples of prompts include to-do lists, grocery lists, daily or weekly pill boxes, cell phone or watch alarms, whiteboard notes, handouts, written or picture instruction sheets, audio or video demonstrations and prompts, and written contracts or agreements. The introduction of new strategies or resources may require support and repetition for integration.

5. Due to common hearing issues, make sure only one person talks at a time when important information is being discussed. Allow time for questions, and always ask me to share back or summarize what was covered. This allows you to make sure I heard and understood what you thought you shared. It also allows me to rehearse the information once, and provides an opportunity to address any missed items, misheard information, or misunderstood concepts.

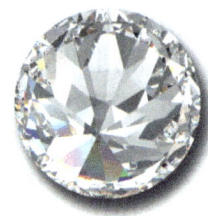

Diamond State

Clear, Sharp, Faceted, Highly Structured

My brain is still clear and sharp, for the most part. I can and do shine much of the time, but at other times I can be cutting or hard, which may not be typical for me at all. I have many facets, so everyone may see me differently, potentially causing conflict among those who know me. As I make mistakes while processing information, I may work to hide the slips-ups, or I may blame the errors on just getting old, being tired, or not focusing. However, when the mistakes happen more frequently, are more intense, or are very uncharacteristic, things might be changing in a more important way. As someone who is supporting me, it will be important to notice and consider frequency, intensity, and patterns over time.

It could be hard to tell if I am just being difficult or stubborn, or if I am truly having changes in my abilities. You may notice I am getting very rigid and inflexible in how I like things, do things, and want things. I may seem less and less aware of boundaries or limits in my expectations. I seem to think I am the center of what is going on and want to be special and unique. Perhaps I seem to care less about others.

I may struggle a lot with changes and new routines, expectations, settings, or situations. I may or may not be aware of these changes. I will want to keep roles, habits, environments, rules, and supports just like they have always been, even if they may no longer be working well for either or both of us.

I also may be more accusatory, thinking that others are trying to trick me or conspire against me. I may be very focused on being frugal with money, finances, and expenses, or conversely, I may spend, gift, and offer money and resources freely to others when I would never have done that before.

I may retain respect for authority figures such as doctors, administrators, lawyers, nurses, rabbis, ministers, law enforcement, and oldest children; or I may seek to discount their power or authority, avoid them, or even disrespect or argue with them.

I may become very angry, anxious, or sad if you try to tell me that I am not functioning as well as I used to, that I am not being logical, or that I am being stubborn, mean, not thinking, or not caring.

It is very possible that people who do not know me well will not be aware of any changes. This is because I may still be skilled at social chit-chat and am usually able to cover for any mistakes during short periods of time. Brief visits in social settings may not allow others to see that I am not able to use some of my higher-level skills in language, empathy, problem solving, way-finding, detailed organization, and new information retention. That said, if I was never very skilled in these areas, the changes or withdrawal from these activities may just seem more like subtle changes and not bigger losses. It is very likely that it is with those I trust the most that I will react the most strongly and adversely.

Even if you know me well, it is possible that you may not notice my changes if you only see me occasionally. At events when I know I need to be at my best, my brain can produce more chemicals and help me function better than I typically do. This may be seen at doctor's appointments, driving tests, and important gatherings. This makes it seem like, during the times when I'm struggling, that I am just not trying; which is not the case, since it is all about brain chemistry.

It is also possible that, even if you are around me frequently, you may not notice how much I am changing because you become accustomed to it. You may become so used to filling in my missing words, reminding me of appointments, or providing other support that you don't even notice when things are changing.

You may notice that I ask the same questions over and over or tell stories repeatedly. Or when I say, "Did I ever tell you ..." you may think, *Only about twenty times!* You may find yourself saying, "Remember, I already told you ..." or "Don't you remember?" This happens because you get tired of hearing it or you become frustrated with my repetition, but for me, it is new information each time.

I may also struggle with finding words at times. I may talk my way around certain words or use vague phrases. Nouns are usually the first words to be missing. I might say, "Where is my ... you know, the thing I use to pay the bills ... ?" when I am looking for my checkbook. I am also beginning to have some trouble with understanding complex phrases and difficulty in keeping up with changes in topics. My speech may seem a little off-target or tangential, or possibly just less frequent.

Helpful Tips for Supporting Someone in a Diamond GEMS State:

1. Recognize the changes and be willing to modify your approach and expectations. When I am in a Diamond State, you need to be the one to change.

2. Stop arguing and give up on trying to orient me to your reality. Let go of needing to be right! Learn how to help and support without being bossy or taking over completely.

3. Be willing to acknowledge problems with an interaction or in the relationship. Try one of these acknowledgments:

- "Whoa! I was trying to help, but what I did was not very helpful!"

- "Wow! It looks like I made you angry." *or* "Wow! It looks like I disappointed you."

- "You are right, that should not have happened."

- "I had no right to make you feel that way or treat you that way."

- "This is hard. I hate this for you." *or* "This is hard. I hate this for us."

4. When I ask or tell you repeatedly about something, stop saying *remember* or *don't you remember?* Instead, use this sequence:

   - Reflect my statement or question back to me to confirm that you heard it.
     - "You want to know what time the appointment is . . ."

   - Offer my answer using a combination of visual and verbal prompts.
     - "It's at three p.m." (show three fingers)

   - Keep your voice and manner calm and friendly, and introduce a new idea.
     - "Oh! Could you help me for a minute?"

   - If you are getting tired or frustrated, take a break or get help. Or, after you respond, try getting me onto another subject or topic by asking for my help, providing something different and interesting to do, or using humor rather than negative emotions to cope.

- "Our appointment is at three p.m." (Show three fingers.) "Oh hey, I could use your help. I need these coupons clipped for the grocery store. Can you do that for me?"

5. Limit advanced sharing of information, appointments, vacations, or plans if this creates distress or anxiety. Post information and reminders if that is helpful for the individual.

   - You don't need to tell me that I have an appointment next month. I may remember that I have an appointment but lose track of the days in between. However, when it is helpful for me to know ahead of time, have helpful reminders where I can see them.

6. Listen to my old stories and learn the details of them, as they will become very helpful as the disease progresses. When I ask, "Did I ever tell you about . . . ?" instead of saying *yes* or *no*, repeat a few of my words back to me and then state, "Tell me about it!" with as much enthusiasm and interest as possible. Keep in mind that I am trying to talk with you, but I want to be in charge of the conversation. I don't remember that I already told you the story, but I am trying hard to connect with you.

7. Let me keep as many old routines and habits as possible. If they aren't working, indicate that an authority figure says we must do something different, at least for now. Emphasize that we need to *try* this, and that it's a rule for everyone. Tell me that you need me to help you out. In other words, it's not about me being incompetent or unable, but about others.

8. Help me establish and maintain a healthy rhythm

to my day, balancing the type of activity between productive, wellness, restorative, and leisure activities. Use environmental and social support to foster this lifestyle and rhythm. Sustain engagement or work to gradually improve the balance. Take it in baby steps!

- And don't forget to look in the mirror and make sure your own day has some balance to it, as well. In this situation, two Diamonds are not better than a Sapphire plus a Diamond.

9. Investigate my safety in independent living skills such as driving or public transportation use, financial management, care of others, medication and health condition management, meals and food management, firearms or power tool/equipment use, or home and car maintenance without having it be confrontational. Consider practicing with a coach to guide you through this process, rather than just winging it.

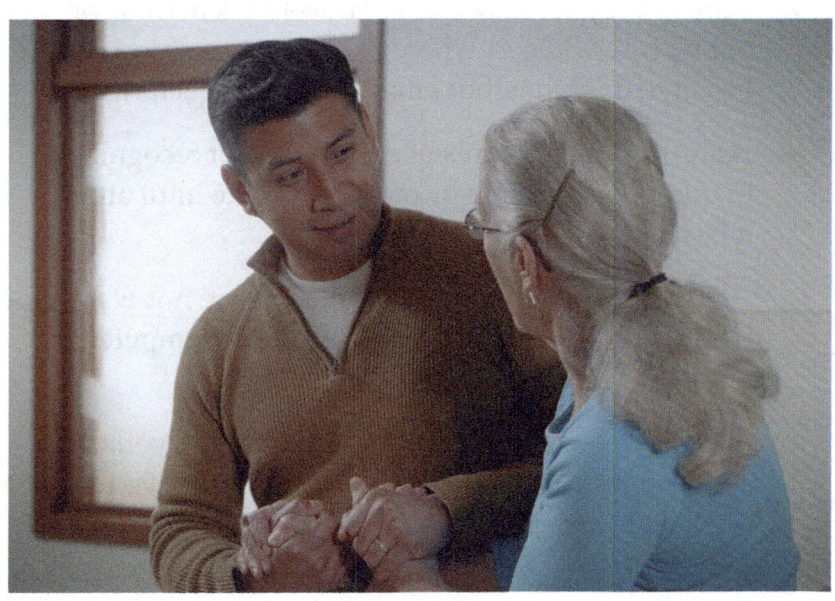

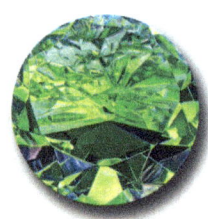

Emerald State

On the Go with Repeating Patterns

As a person spends more time in an Emerald State, this is often when a diagnosis is received. It becomes harder to brush aside the mistakes and changes we notice as being due to other factors and we become more curious as to what else could be going on.

The Emerald State is where we'll start to see a person's awareness and ability be widely variable.

- In this state, I may have limited awareness, no awareness, or hyperintense awareness of my ability changes.

- I am on the go: I may seem to travel back in time, or not be sure when or where I am going somewhere. I want to do things, but I may struggle to get it right.

- I can and will make mistakes but may not recognize that I am responsible or made a mistake until after it has happened.

    o Even though I make mistakes, I may not want you to help me if it makes me feel incompetent or stupid.

    o I will resent being treated like a child if you try to physically assist or help, or if you give too much information for me to handle at that moment.

- - This may result in an explosion of emotion or a need to get away from you or the situation, or an emotional collapse and sense of intense failure.
- If I am feeling unsure about my skills, I may prefer to watch or supervise you, rather than doing it myself.
- I pay more attention to what I *see* than what I *hear* when I am in an Emerald State.
  - If I don't see something, I often miss it altogether.
- I may skip a personal care routine, thinking I already did it today, when in fact it was yesterday or last week when I actually did it.
  - Conversely, I may do a task over and over in a single day.
- When I am tired, stressed, or ill, my changes are more noticeable:
  - shorter cycles on repeats.
  - more emotionally fragile.
  - needing more cues and support to make life doable.

Vision Changes

In this state, my functional vision is mostly binocular, with limited peripheral awareness around the edges of my visual field. It's important to realize I have not actually lost the vision in my visual field. My eyes are working as they always have, but my brain is just not able to take in and process all the data. It selects what seems most important at the moment, which may result in intense focus in the center of my field or scanning around in a disorganized fashion to try to locate the object of value.

Because of this, I lack awareness of what is to the sides, down low, and up high. I might miss objects that are right in front of me, such as my food, my glasses, or the phone, because I am focusing on something else. If I am looking for something, I may scan all over but still not actually *see* it.

To get a better idea of what I can see in this State, make circles with your hands and put them over your eyes as if they were binoculars. Notice what you can see and what you can't, particularly on your body.

Time and Place

If I am living with dementia, I may think I am in a different time and place in my life, especially later in the day, if I am stressed or ill, or if I am in an unfamiliar place such as a hospital or a friend's house. During these periods, I may not recognize your relation to me.

- For example, I may think my children are still young, so rather than recognizing someone as my grown daughter, I may think they are a friend or even my mother.

- I may not recognize the person I have been married to for fifty years because I am looking for the man from my wedding photo.

- I may think I am very young and may start looking for my childhood home, insisting that I am not at home.

- In these moments, I may think strangers are friends, and friends are strangers. I don't mean to hurt you, but I am lost in my life in these moments and am seeking safety or adventure.

Language and Communication

When I am in an Emerald State, you may notice a change in my language and communication skills. This is generally due to the areas in the brain that are being affected by my dementia.

- My left temporal lobe, which is where my vocabulary, language comprehension, and speech production skills are located, is often impacted by dementia.
    - I can chit-chat, but I may start to struggle with losing nouns, using vague language, misspeaking, describing a word instead of remembering it, or using visual cues rather than saying what I want to say.
    - I might miss one-fourth of the words in a sentence.
    - When you try to explain something or reason with me, I may become upset.
    - Even if I am not getting all the words, I can tell when you are not happy with me by your tone of voice and facial expression.
    - I may initially agree to do something, only to feel tricked and refuse when I figure out what you actually meant. This is because I may not have fully understood what you were asking me to do or I don't like the way you are doing something.

Emotions, Time of Day

In human brains, the prefrontal cortex is an area that does not fully develop until young adulthood. One of its jobs is to regulate our primitive brain, which is responsible for the:

- Fright, flight, or fight response.

- Seeking of pleasure.
- Meeting of needs.

In an Emerald State, there are a few reasons why my prefrontal cortex may not be working as well. I may be fatigued, needing fuel, or experiencing changing abilities due to dementia—or a combination of all of these.

When this happens, you may see:

- My emotions may get out of control easily, usually more so in the later afternoons or evenings when I am worn out.
- I may become restless as I seek a place of familiarity or comfort.
- I may really enjoy events but struggle afterward due to fatigue and depletion of my brain chemicals.

Confabulation

When I am struggling to remember something, my brain may try to fill in the blank spots with false memories, which is known as **confabulation**. This makes it seem as if I am making things up or lying to *you*, but my *brain* is actually lying to *me*.

If you try to argue with me about it, I will tend to become more suspicious, resentful, and fearful, making care interactions much more challenging. I generally can remember strong feelings toward you or others, but I won't always remember the details of why I feel that way. So, my brain will make up information to help it make sense to me—I often can't be logical or rational about it. So, if you try to get me to *get it*, we will have conflict.

Time Use and a Feeling of Discomfort

I likely struggle with time use and may continually seek guidance, asking, "What do I do now? Where should I go?"

- I may just stay in my familiar, comfortable location and not want to do much or venture out.
- Conversely, I might have a high risk of eloping or seeking out different places, situations, or people, resulting in the need for search and rescue assistance.

Skills and (In)dependence

Another factor that can be at either end of the spectrum is my confidence in my own skills. I will likely either think I am more competent than I am, or seek out constant guidance, reassurance, and help. Both extremes will wear on you.

- Overestimation of my skills and abilities will result in changes in the quality of my personal care routines and appearance. It can also result in problems with personal hygiene, unsafe task performance, and major issues with managing other health conditions.
- On the other hand, constant reassurance will tire you, as I am unable to hold onto things that we just did or the information you told me. I may constantly seek to be close to you to shadow you, and I may worry if you are out of my sight.

Helpful Tips for Supporting Someone in an Emerald GEMS State:

1. Learn the importance of asking yourself, *so what?* before deciding to act. If I have made an error or I am doing something that is new or different, stop and consider: do you really need to do something about this right now? Will it matter in five minutes,

five days, five months, or five years? Is it worth the damage it may cause to our relationship? Learn the difference between something that is simply annoying and something that is truly risky or dangerous for me or others. Can it wait for a bit, and you can retry in a while? Can you reconsider your options?

2. Greet before you treat! Learn the importance of getting connected to me and establishing a relationship every time. This is especially true before you try to address or fix something that I did in error. Consider offering information about yourself rather than assuming that I can or cannot recognize you. Try, "Hey, it's Teepa!" as a greeting—but remember to use your name, not mine.

3. Learn how to do things *with* me, not *to* me or *for* me. Let me be a partner and feel that we are in this together.

4. If I am lost in time, accept that at this moment I may be focused on an episode from before. I may be in a different time and place. I need you to stay calm, get connected in a way I can understand, listen to me, try to figure out what I need, and work to meet that need. Instead of trying to get me to understand reality as you know it, try this instead:

    - Offer your name in greeting. You may need to use my name rather than our relationship. For example, "Hi, Mary, it's John" *rather than* "Hi, Mom, it's me."

    - If I don't seem to know who you are to me, let it go. Be okay with being a friend instead of a family member or being a different family member.

- If I say, "I want to go home," or "I'm looking for my mother," don't argue or use reality orientation. Instead:
    o Get connected using the Positive Physical Approach (see page 55).
    o Reflect my words back to me, using a question rhythm to confirm what is being asked: "You need to get home...?" *or* "You want to find your mother...?"
- Then, make an emotionally supportive comment such as: "You have always loved being at home..." *or* "Sounds like you are really missing your mother." Pause and listen to how I respond.
- If my language abilities allow, say, "Tell me about your home" *or* "Tell me about your mother."
- If language is a challenge for me, ask specific information about the place or person, such as :
    o "You have something you need to do at home, or do you just want to be there?"
    o "Is your mother a great cook, or not so good? Do you like her dinners or desserts better?"
- Use reflection when the person provides you with information.
- Match the number of words or phrases that the person is using to stay connected with them. For instance, if they are using only four to five words at a time, then you do the same.

- It could be that something about the environment is causing me to seek a place or person. Consider taking me for a walk or a ride to a more unfamiliar place for a short time. When I return, I may reconnect with the location and feel okay.

5. When you want me to do something, use visual cues such as gestures, props, or demonstrations first. Do actions alongside me on my dominant side, not *to* me.

6. Think before you speak:

    - Limit how much you say and pause after each sentence. Slow it down a little and wait for my responses.

    - Make sure your visual cues, including your facial expressions, match your verbal information. Show, then tell.

    - When you change subjects or topics, give a strong visual and verbal cue of the switch.
        - For example, you might gesture and say *Oh!* as if you were remembering something new you were going to say.

    - Notice things out loud and with gestures:
        - For example, "Isn't that interesting?!" while pointing to a nearby object.

    - Offer me either/or choices, like:
        - "Would you like something hot or cold to drink?" rather than open-ended questions like, "What do you want to drink?"

    - If I say, "I need something," respond with:

- - "You need something?" Pause, then add, "Tell me more about it" *or* "Could you show me what you do with it?"
  - Please don't ask me what I need. I'm very likely having trouble finding the words.
- Build a daily routine and schedule that provides regular structure and sequence.
  - Be careful about special events and surprises—keep them small, simple, and short, and be willing to let it go if it is not going well.

7. If what you want is not working, pause and back off, change something, and then reapproach and try again.

8. You will need to learn how to *respond*, rather than *react*, to what I do or say. It may feel like work at times. Think it through and try to appreciate the true meaning before trying to fix something, explain something, or change something!

9. Use humor, but laugh *with* me, not *at* me. If I don't find it funny, stop and acknowledge how I might be feeling or what is happening for me. Be willing to laugh at yourself about mistakes you make in front of me. Being imperfect is an art form! *Oops* moments may create universal connections. Haven't we all had *uh-ohs* at one time or another?

10. Break tasks, activities, and expectations down into smaller steps. Help me want to get up and get going before you talk about details of personal care or other items that need to happen. Try to think about what I would like to do, not what needs to be done.

11. Ask if I can help you, rather than telling me that you

need or want to help me. Help me feel like I still matter and make a difference. Share tasks with me, don't do *for* me or try to do *to* me. If I ask what I can do to help, have a few options ready, and consider offering a *this or that* option.

12. Consider writing out a first-person narrative of my life story and share key pieces of information with others involved in my care. When others understand my history and life experiences, they can better support me.

13. If you are aware of them, share information about my preferences and personality. It is helpful to know whether I am a risk taker or safety seeker, if I am introverted or extroverted, my likes/dislikes, and preferred types of activities. This will help team members know how to help build a day that works well for me.

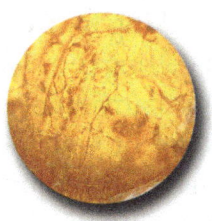

Amber State

Caution Light, Caught in a Moment of Time

In the Amber State, I am caught in a moment and focused on the sensation or the experience. If it seems as if I am stuck, you will need to wait and attempt to get my attention again in a short while. During tasks, I may need you to stop and give me a break, or I might become verbally or physically distressed. Although I may not always be focused on your relationship with me, I will typically know whether or not I like you based on how you look, sound, move, smell, or respond.

When dementia is involved and my actions are not typical of what I used to do before and are often based on my sensory preferences of the moment, it may be more challenging for you to spend time with me. It may surprise you when I investigate, touch, handle, smell, taste, or take apart objects, or otherwise engage the way I do. It is a function of how my brain is currently processing incoming data and providing me with input. I may also overreact or underreact to various situations.

When I am in an Amber State, I have limited safety awareness and don't understand much of the *why* behind what you are trying to get me to do or not do. I want what I want and like. What I don't like or can't tolerate, I won't do. I often have very limited tolerance for waiting—you will need to respond to me as soon as possible! And yet you may have to wait for me to be ready and willing.

I may seem very self-focused, because my brain is seeking out sensations it likes and working to avoid what it doesn't like. I may not be aware if I am getting too close to other individuals, taking others' belongings, damaging objects, or hurting your feelings, as I am less aware of your needs and expectations. However, I still want to have fun, enjoy myself, get connected, do my own thing, and meet my needs.

I may at times not remember what certain objects are or how to use them. Please secure spaces and items that could harm me or cause significant damage. This also means I may not understand the purpose of things, but you should continue to provide me with plenty of items I can interact with, use, and enjoy.

Exercising my hand-eye coordination skills is very important, as it will help me maintain my dexterity as long as possible. It will allow me to practice and use brain circuitry that connects sensation with motor control. The value of what I am doing is in the *doing*, not in the end result. I may want and need to do things over and over at times. These experiences should be based on what I am enjoying and engaging with, not necessarily on what I have done before. Simple sorting or manipulative tasks may seem too easy, but they help me feel skilled and competent.

I may not be able to tolerate some personal care routines that I once thought were essential to me. This is largely based on how my brain is handling sensory data. Typically, five areas of my body may become more sensitive:

- the lips/tongue/mouth area
- the palms of the hands and fingertips
- the armpits
- the soles of the feet and toes
- genitalia

Care activities involving these areas may distress me, including activities such as taking pills, shaving or facial hair removal, mouth and denture care, eating and drinking, hand washing and nail care, foot care, and toileting. If something doesn't seem to be going well, back off and reapproach in just a few minutes. Although I am hypersensitive in these areas, I am often not as aware of other parts of my body. This means I do not always feel what is wrong or pick up on my body's cues. I may have issues with incontinence or not be aware when I am hungry, thirsty, tired, hurting, or too hot or cold.

To get a sense of how this might feel for those of us living with healthy brains, consider this scenario: You are at a crowded party, enjoying some chips and dip. Then suddenly, a person nearby unexpectedly leans over and wipes dip off the corner of your mouth with a napkin. They noticed that it was about to drip onto your shirt, and you didn't happen to have a napkin in your hand. *Whoa!* That would be a sensory surprise, and probably a bit unwelcome. At that moment, it is highly likely that you might enter an Amber State of mind.

Helpful Tips for Supporting Someone in an Amber GEMS State:

1. Use my actions to guide your responses. Be prepared for changes in my sensory needs and tolerance issues. Plan to keep visits short if it is hard to be with me. It is better to have five good minutes than an hour of distress.

2. Look. Listen. Feel. Smell. Taste. Be curious about the sensations I am seeking, avoiding, wanting, or disliking, and then try to either help me get what I want or reduce what is bothering me.

3. Sometimes the best thing to do is take a pause, a time-out. Step away for a few minutes, breathe deeply and completely, then try to reapproach and reconnect using Visual-Verbal-Touch cues that seem to match what I am doing.

- Visual-Verbal-Touch (V-V-T) is the order in which I process information best.
    - Visual—Show me what you want me to pay attention to.
    - Verbal—Using only a few words at a time.
    - Touch—Only with my permission, preferably using Hand-under-Hand.
- If you communicate with me in this order, I am much less likely to resist or become distressed.

4. Notice my pace. Be willing to slow down or speed up to match me first, then gradually change the rhythm and pattern to reach a more comfortable level. This will be more effective than trying to get me to stop or get going.

5. Create a list of my sensory experiences and past preferences based on what you have noticed and observed. Get input from others, if possible, as well.
    - What I like to look at and explore visually: any types of pictures, videos, or sight-based items I seem to really connect with.
    - What I like to hear: musical and auditory preferences, volume preferences, any accent or speech factors that seem to make a difference.
    - What touch and movement sensations I like and what I seem to avoid: being touched versus touching, types of textures and temperatures (for food and drink as well as handling), space from others, speed of movement, or rhythmic actions or movements such as dancing, walking, exercising, rocking, or swaying.
    - Olfactory stimulation (smells) that calm or

stimulate me, as well as smells that I dislike or am sensitive to.

- Taste preferences for food and drink, including favorite flavors, seasonings/spices, and recipes; and items I dislike.

6. It will be important to simplify my world, tasks, expectations, and interactions. Simplify, but don't *babify*. Don't infantilize or treat me as if I am stupid, just simplify.

7. When greeting me and offering me cues, exaggerate visual responses, use automatic social greetings and gestures, limit verbal information and instructions, and use Hand-under-Hand and Visual-Verbal-Touch guidance and assistance (see pages 45 and 55 for details). Support me, rather than doing things *to* me or *for* me.

8. Eating when there is a lack of object recognition can look like *playing* with my food or making a mess. Consider offering just one food item at a time and use demonstration and Hand-under-Hand to get the activity started or to switch from eating to drinking and vice versa.

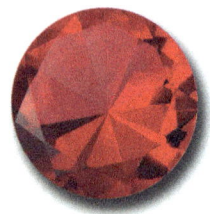

Ruby State

Red Light on Skills, Hidden Depths

The Ruby State is all about big motions with repeated actions, or being still and static. In this state, I may feel that I need to walk, jog, dance, knead dough, or beat a drum. I am in the rhythm pattern. It could be that I am gazing at something that catches my eye, listening to something that catches my ear, or stroking or rocking with a repeating motion that is calming or energizing. I am not aware of the details of the world around me, only my own personal experience at that moment.

With dementia, my brain is trying hard to work, but it is struggling to understand the world around me. I still have deep, rich moments, but they are fewer and harder to see from your perspective. My fine motor skills and detailed abilities are failing, but my big movements and automatic actions, words, and reactions are frequently still present.

Changing gears or transitioning activities too quickly may result in a red light for me. I am more likely to repeat what I am doing than switch to doing something new. If you want me to switch, please use clear, strong visual plus audio cues first, then touch and movement cues that help me make the shift (V-V-T). I am slowing down in all areas of ability, so if you try to get me to go too fast, I am likely to shut down, resist, try to get away from you, or become frightened and immobilized. Alternatively, I might demonstrate fast, powerful, and surprisingly skilled movements when I get into a rhythm.

I still have some automatic speech and some rhythm to my speech. I can pick up your rhythms in speech and can generally still sing or hum along. I may dance much better than I can walk.

My fine motor skills are changing in several areas:

1. I am losing fine motor control in my eye function while keeping general vision skills. My vision is changing to becoming monocular: my brain can no longer take the data that is coming in through each eye and process it so that I am able to see three-dimensional images.

    - Remember in the Emerald State (see page 10) I mentioned that you could create circles with your hands to go over both eyes? Those were binoculars. In this GEMS State, we are at a monocular ability. So close one eye, keep your hand circle over the open eye, and notice the difference.

2. As a result, I may have double vision or ignore one image so the other is clear.

    - Typically, I lack depth perception. I misjudge distances, such as thinking an object is closer than it is.

    - I may see a pattern in the carpet and think it is something to be picked up, think that a change in flooring is a step, or feel that a doorway is a hole or too small to get through.

    - I am also often not aware that there is a bigger world other than what I see. This means I can get stuck in corners, behind doors, or in a room, and not know how to get out.

    - I can also trip over large objects and anything in my path that I don't notice when I am moving toward something I want or like.

    - When I don't see something, I will not know it exists. So, when I turn around to sit down, I may not see that there is a chair behind me, and start walking again, still looking for a place to sit.

3. I am losing my fine motor skills in my hands and fingers.

    - I tend to hold, take, carry, wipe, grasp, or pinch with my thumb rather than use my fingers to manipulate items.

    - I do not have good judgment on my grip strength, and if I am looking at something else, I may forget I have something in my hand.

    - I am losing the ability to use utensils and tools and complete bilateral fine motor tasks such as buttoning, zipping, spearing with a fork, or using a toothbrush skillfully on my own.

4. I am losing fine motor control in my feet and toes, but I am keeping my big movements. I may have either a constant desire to move or I may develop an intense fear of falling due to a lack of balance and coordination.

    - Immobility may increase due to my fear of falling because I know I am unstable.

    - I am often able to do automatic movements and actions, but if I think about it or must plan it out, I have more difficulty. I get stuck easily when I can't figure out what to do or how to do it.

    - Pulling or pushing me (such as when I forget the chair is there and I am about to sit down) is very scary and it feels like you are trying to make me fall or hurt me, so I may react strongly and swiftly.

5. I am losing fine motor skill in my lips, tongue, and mouth. I can suck and swallow, either take a bite or a drink, but if it is mixed (soup with chunks, big

bites of food with drinks), I may either take in only the liquid or only the solid items. I am more likely to aspirate than before.

- I may also accidentally hold food in my cheeks, known as pocketing, as I am less aware of the sides of my mouth and can't control those muscles as well.

- I may also suck on an item that is hard to manage. I may spit it back out or hold it in my mouth because I'm not sure what to do with it.

In addition to the loss of fine motor skills, I am less aware of my physical self and the incoming sensory information from most of my body and organ systems. At the same time, there are some body locations that become hypersensitized. I feel strongly in these areas and may overreact when they are touched. These areas are my lips, tongue, and mouth (especially right in the front), my fingertips and fingernails, the soles of my feet and toes, my armpits, and my genital area.

There may be many situations when I am less interested in eating meals. I may graze more than sit down and eat a whole meal, so I tend to lose weight. I may be burning calories faster or having more trouble eating. There is also a possibility that my internal absorption of nourishment is being affected by my brain changes. Watch for signs and signals of hunger or thirst in my behavior, as I generally am not aware of what I am feeling and won't be able to tell you. At the same time, be aware that more is not necessarily better, as I may have trouble processing all that is consumed. My digestive tract's inconsistent abilities may result in episodes of constipation and loose stools.

If I get injured, I might not seem to be aware of it. Since I have limited body awareness, I don't know where or what is bothering me, so I might just seem more irritated or agitated, or more somnolent and less alert and aware.

Everything is slowing down, and I can only handle limited stimulation. It takes longer for me to process information, so I need you to slow down and break things down into smaller bits.

Be prepared for the possibility of more short periods of rest or sleep rather than one long nighttime sleep period. Some dementias make deep, refreshing sleep difficult to achieve.

Helpful Tips for Supporting Someone in a Ruby GEMS State:

- Use my given name with a positive and energizing tone to get my attention. Avoid repeating my name over and over or using a voice that indicates disapproval or frustration.

- Slow down: it takes me longer to figure things out, do things, process anything, or react.

- Use my automatic skills when possible, such as rhythm, music, greetings, rhymes, poetry, or movements. Avoid details or specifics that I have to copy to initiate, select, or sequence.

- Break tasks down into small steps. You will need to think it through before you get started. First, determine where you want to end up, but remember to present only one step at a time for me (see Teepa's PIPES and 5Ps on page 74 and 75).

- Work on demonstrating and showing me what you want me to do, rather than telling me using words.

- Start where I am, and then gradually shift gears until you help me get to the new state of motion or activity desired.

- Plan my day to have a balance of restful and active periods, and plan to help me transition slowly and gradually from one to the other.

- Manage the sensory and physical environment for calming or stimulating cues, depending on what I need at that time.

- Use Hand-under-Hand® (HuH) for mobility support. To let me know where to go or what to notice, point with your other hand while in Hand-under-Hand (see page 45 for more information on HuH).

- Guide and cue, don't push, pull, or use force. The more you push me, verbally or physically, the more likely it is that I will react and/or resist.

- Use Hand-under-Hand to touch and provide care, as it provides my brain with more information and reduces sensitivity responses in key care areas as I am used to me touching me.

- Use your voice to engage and encourage, but limit talking. This is especially true if I am trying to move away from you, or we are in a noisy space or participating in a busy activity. Be willing to be silent with me.

- Use what is calming to me and my senses to help me settle. Use what is stimulating to help me get going again. Think in shorter windows of active or passive engagement with longer transitions to shift from one thing/place/person/prop/program to another. Or try to have two possibilities in mind, so you don't hit a dead end with a refusal.

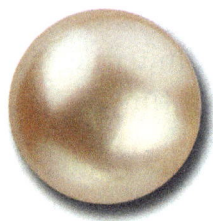

Pearl State

Hidden Within a Shell, Quiet Beauty

Imagine yourself when you are asleep. You are in your body and yet you are not aware of much, either within yourself, or the world around you. This is an example of the Pearl State. Those who meditate may recognize this experience of being inside yourself and relatively unaware of what is taking place around you. In a Pearl State, you can notice voices or contacts. People who approach quietly, calmly, slowly, and with a stable touch tend to bring a person out of themselves in a way that is comfortable. Conversely, loud, demanding voices, or quick, intrusive touch can startle, irritate, or cause an intense reaction.

With dementia, the brain is losing its ability to guide and direct my body. The control system for moving, interacting, processing, and responding is failing. I am still here, but I am getting ready to leave. Just like an oyster in a shell, I am hidden inside the shell of my body. Much of what my body does is ruled by reflexes. My muscles tend to be active and turned on most of the time, so I have a higher risk of contracture formation, where my limbs are curled inward. This cannot be fixed with casting or braces. I may startle easily and tighten up even more with quick movements, loud sounds, changes in light, unexpected touch, etc. My balance is very limited, and I may not be aware of leaning or sitting in one position for a long time.

I am struggling to understand what you say. If you only use words and get loud, I may shut down and retreat. I tend to respond best to familiar voices, rhythms, touches, and gradual, gentle, firm movements. Let me know you are there and that you are going to help me move, and then gradually reposition me.

Please don't think that because I am not awake and alert, it is better to just hurry and get a task over with as quickly as possible.

In this state, my internal systems are starting to malfunction much of the time, as well. I am not very interested in food or drink, and I am starting to have trouble with coordinating swallowing and breathing. Helping me eat is a slow process and can be hard. I might not want more, and yet you recognize that if I don't take in more food or drink, I will become dehydrated and malnourished. If you try to get me to take in what I can't manage, I can aspirate—when food or drink goes into my lungs rather than into my stomach. Even when I do take in these items, I may not be able to get them to go into the right place. Just because I am not coughing, it doesn't mean I am swallowing effectively. Sometimes my brain can't recognize the problem, so it doesn't react. This means I may develop pneumonia and be unable to fight it because my immune system is also failing.

It is important to remember that it is normal for me to have muscle wasting and weight loss when I am spending a lot of time in this state. I may develop wounds that don't heal because I don't have enough protein for the healing process. I am very prone to infections because my brain doesn't recognize and organize a response to them.

It is critical to work through your grief to accept that my condition may well be terminal. The things you are seeing may be just the symptoms of the end of the disease. All my body systems are failing. Your efforts to try to hang on to me by fixing bits and pieces will not change the big picture. The gift is that my body and brain are preparing for this. As I eat and drink less and less, my brain releases endorphins. This allows me to not be distressed or in pain. I will not be hungry or thirsty when this happens. If you are ready, you may be able to offer me the greatest gift of all: letting me know it is all right to go. I may not be able to leave you easily without your permission. After all, inside this shell, I still care and have moments when I can process and respond.

Even though I spend much of the time resting or seeming unaware of the world around me, there will be moments when I become alert and responsive. At these times, the shell opens, and you can see me, the pearl, shining through.

Helpful Tips for Supporting
Someone in a Pearl GEMS State:

1. Take time to observe me before approaching.

2. If I am not alert, use your voice and touch in a friendly and rhythmic way to bring me back to alertness and awareness.

3. If I am present, use the moment to connect and interact with me, using sequential multimodal cues of sight, sound, touch, smell, and possibly taste. Go slow and give me time to take in information, process it, and then respond.

4. Use the time we are together to be with me, not just care for me.

5. Always keep one still hand on my shoulder, hip, hand, or back when you are doing something with the other hand. That way, I have a better sense of where you are, and I don't lose you.

6. Consider body experiences to allow me to have time that I can enjoy, such as cuddling close, stroking a pet, feeling the sun or a breeze on my face, or hearing sounds such as deep chimes, chants, favorite prayers, poems, or readings. Use smells that I seem to enjoy, modeling how to sniff deeply to help me know what to do.

7. Offer me sips and tastes but be less concerned about getting me to eat or drink. It should be about what I like, not about what is good for me at this point in the journey.

8. Talk to me and with me just as if I were sitting right there with you, because I am. Please don't talk about me as though I am an object or as if I'm not here.

9. Create opportunities for me to engage and respond, but don't force it or expect it. I am doing the best I can.

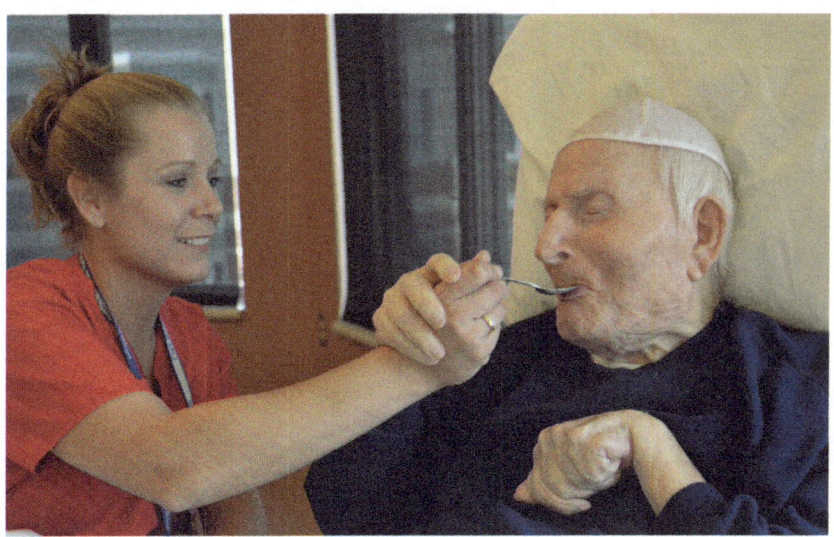

GEMS® State Support to Consider

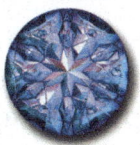

Sapphire State

- Take breaks for self-care.
- Build in opportunities for rest and restoration.
- Discover what you like about the person or people you support.
- Find support that works for you to find purpose, joy, and satisfaction each day.

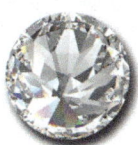

Diamond State

- Daily/weekly check-ins for health issues that are changing or are critical, such as a new diagnosis, change in medication, or new treatment regimen.
- System to monitor finances, medications, transportation, pet or spouse care, and environmental safety.
- Notification of events in a way that matches the person's need to know and ability to hold onto the information. Slightly in advance or just before the event is typically most effective.
- Interactions that help the individual feel special, valued, and engaged.

- May need a family meeting with a skilled facilitator to help everyone understand the situation and create a plan of support and care that addresses places, people, props/objects, programming, and some possibilities.

- Consider the value of planning for the probable future while the person can actively participate. It is important to not push the agenda, yet appreciate the possibility of a need for change over time and a determination of a better way of beginning that process in small steps.

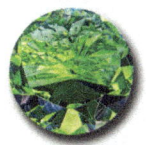

Emerald State

- Daily structure, and consider that more support and guidance may be needed in the afternoon and evening due to brain fatigue and the individual feeling increased distress about where they think they are or should be.

- Items that look and feel right and are familiar to the individual.

- Balance of productive, self-care, leisure, and restorative programming each day. Someone in an Emerald State has difficulty planning out or putting together a whole balanced day without support.

- Use visual cues first and then verbal information, making sure to match the visual to verbal and check for comprehension.

- Touching should be done with permission and should be friendly, not forced.

- Having more than one care partner who is intimately familiar with the preferences and habits of the person is strongly recommended to allow for breaks, variety, and well-being of all.

- Consider a secured or more closely monitored care location if and when the person physically tries to go to another time or place. The best predictor of elopement/wandering is having done it before combined with a life history of exploration or strong patterns of movement through various physical environments throughout a day.

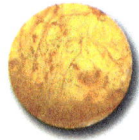

Amber State

- Continuous visual monitoring for safety and engagement with frequent interjections, physical guidance, and cueing assistance to complete care tasks.

- Guiding, directing, stimulating interest, or reducing distress will be needed for maximal safety. The challenge is whether this level of interaction will be tolerated without seeking to remove the person or themselves. It is possible that technology may be needed as a substitute for personnel due to financial or personal limitations or demands.

- An environment that is protective and yet provides positive stimulation and experiences will be essential.

- Each interaction will provide opportunities to consider task or environmental substitutions for better future interactions and safety considerations.

- Personnel and care partners who are alert to the individual's needs and interests and respond quickly and effectively, without being judgmental or parental.

- Care partners who want to be with the individual and can guide and redirect, stop and retry later, interpret nonverbal cues and behaviors, and know how to take time-outs when they need breaks rather than become frustrated with the individual.

- Programming that provides smooth transitions from stimulation to relaxation and back throughout the day and into the evening, and possibly at night, as well, if there is nighttime wakefulness.

- A team of care partners is needed, so that everyone can get rest and be ready to help the individual, who is typically only able to be in the present moment without caution or much safety awareness, but possibly great curiosity.

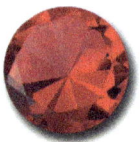

Ruby State

- Continuous availability of physical assistance, supervision, and programming to meet the increasing physical care needs and safety concerns in any environment.

- May require two care partners at times to support with movement and/or personal care: one to focus on the person and their needs and effort to communicate or react, and one to support and help manage the task and environment.

- Daily routines are structured but flexible, and based on the individual's rhythm of wake and sleep.

- Extra time and assistance needed in transitioning from active to quiet, and quiet to active activities.

- Spaces and supports that allow and encourage the right amount of movement and mobility, but are protective and limited, to create safer options that foster retained ability use.

- Sensory-rich environments that use the individual's background and preferences to create opportunities for sights, sounds, textures, temperatures, movements, smells, and tastes of interest and enjoyment.

- Environments, objects, and people that can stimulate or calm, depending on what is needed at the time.

- Individualized engagement opportunities that are balanced and provided in places and spaces that create a sense of security, familiarity, and acceptance.

- Willingness to accept that falls and loss of balance

will probably happen, despite all efforts. A more reasonable goal is to try to minimize fall-related injuries rather than prevent the risk of any fall.

- Willingness to accept that weight loss is an indicator of changing brain abilities rather than a failure to provide enough food or drink. A more reasonable goal is to encourage intake with support as it is tolerated and enjoyed by the person.

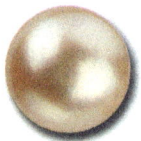

Pearl State

- Continuous supportive monitoring that does not startle, distress, disrupt, or disturb, for needs and care provision.

- Physical care throughout a twenty-four-hour period as needed and tolerated.

- Responsive care that uses nonverbal cues to guide what is done and how it is done.

- Specialized seating and sleeping options, based on postures and contractures.

- Sensory-rich environment that provides sensation that comforts and stimulates on an individualized routine.

- Places, spaces, and opportunities that encourage whatever participation is possible, without demanding more than is desired or needed.

- Modification of routines as conditions shift and change, and a willingness to let go of old habits to accept what seems right for this situation at this moment.

Hand-under-Hand® Support

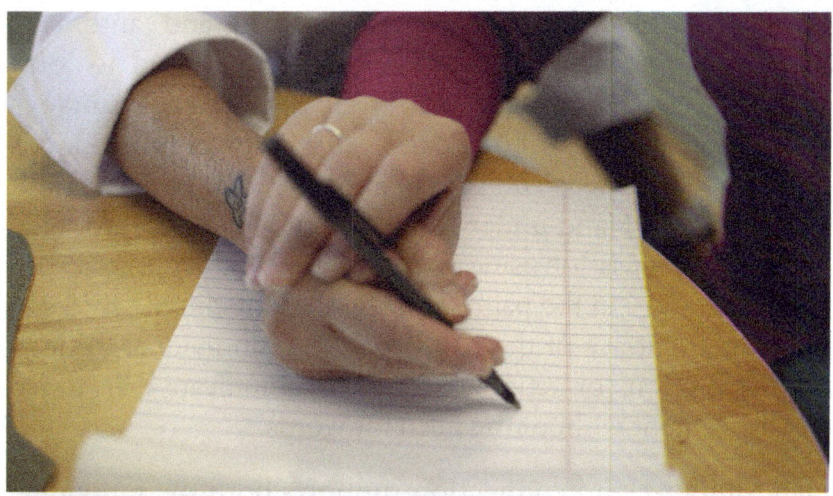

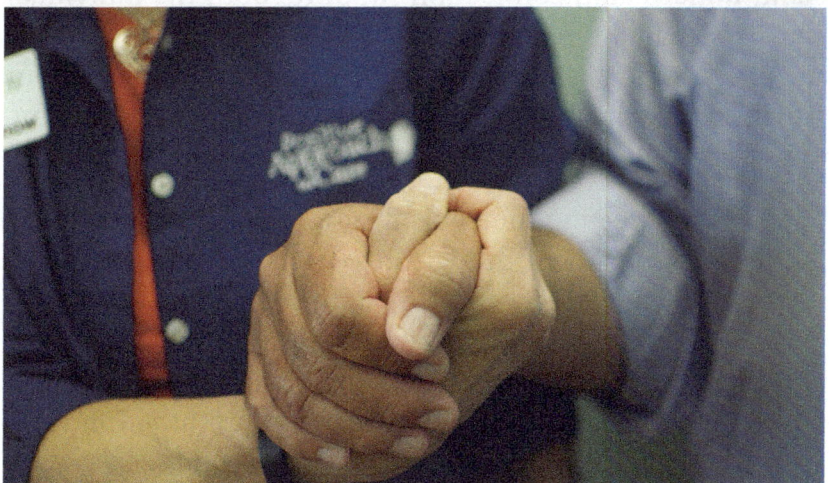

This guidance and assisting technique is an essential support tool for care partners. It provides a strong neurological and familiar connection between two individuals. It also offers the potential of protection for both parties if the guidance or assistance being offered is not wanted. Hand-under-Hand allows a physical touch that is friendly, comforting, and attention-getting without being intrusive or overbearing.

It also provides a system of feedback and communication between the person living with brain change and the person who is supporting them, when tasks, environments, or situations are challenging.

Hand-under-Hand uses the well-practiced and automatic connection between an individual's eye and hand to form a closed circuit between two individuals. The hand-eye connection is one of the very first sensorimotor loops established in infants and is used almost endlessly throughout our daily lives. Hand-under-Hand also provides a comfortable and calming sensation using a familiar grasp and proprioception (deep pressure) in the palm at the base of the thumb. By using the palmar surface of the hand to take an individual through desired motions or actions, we can communicate with touch and movement without the need for words.

Hand-under-Hand connection supports both the individual who is struggling to understand words, tasks, and objects, and the care partner who knows what should be done but struggles to help the individual understand. Here are some ways that Hand-under-Hand can be used:

1. When greeting someone, it sustains a physical connection, allowing the person to be more comfortable with your presence in their intimate space (within arm's reach). Having a comfortable handhold makes it easier to be close. It is very different than a normal handshake that can be uncomfortable to sustain and typically feels awkward after a few seconds. When using a Hand-under-Hand position, you can tell if the person is enjoying your presence or if they want more space without having them become distressed or upset. If they keep trying to let go of your hand, release the position and move back a little farther. They may need a break or may not want you in their intimate space at that moment.

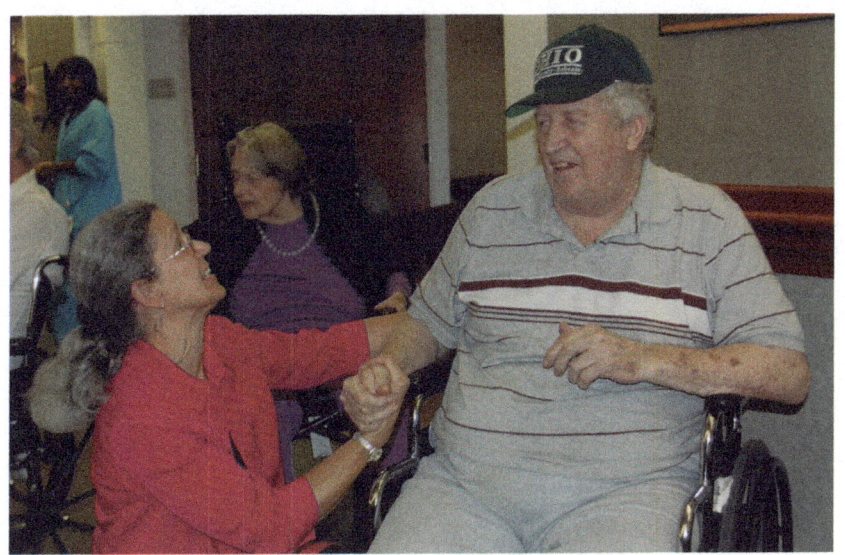

2. It can be used to assist someone with movement. Hand-under-Hand provides effective stability and support, as well as a feedback loop. Since the arm of the person being supported is like the rudder that guides a ship, gently rotating the forearm outward or inward can direct their walking path. By tipping their forearm down, we can indicate physically the cue to sit down in a chair, on the commode, or on the bed. By tipping the forearm slightly upward, we can help the person stand more upright, getting their spine aligned and over their base of support. When used in combination with a gesture of pointing, it can help provide direction and reassurance when mobility is a challenge, when the setting is unfamiliar, or when surfaces are uneven. Because the care partner and individual are close to one another, it is easy to perceive and respond quickly to issues with balance, coordination, fear, or distress. Knowing the person's dominant hand and using that side for Hand-under-Hand support is especially important in accessing procedural memories, old habits and routines, and familiar

patterns of movements that trigger the next steps in sequences.

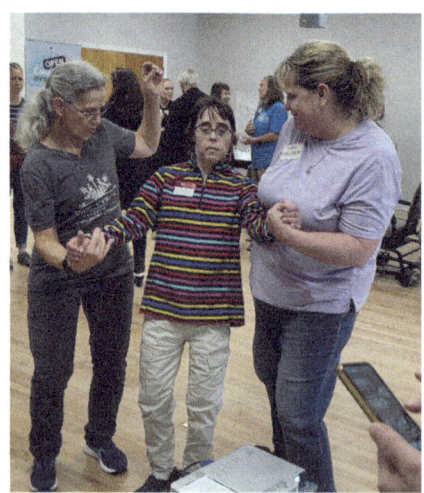

3. Hand-under-Hand is essential when someone is in an Amber, Ruby, or Pearl GEMS State. It provides the care partner a way to help the individual understand the action being requested. It also enables the care partner to use their own dexterity to manipulate a tool or utensil while the person living with brain change still actively participates. This is particularly helpful in motions from hand to mouth, hand to chest, or hand to intimate body parts (armpits and perineal areas), which they have done their entire lives. This automatic loop allows people living with dementia a sense of both control and involvement. It provides the helper with a way to get feedback on preferences, understanding, readiness, and willingness to participate. It provides a way to do *with*, not do *to* or do *for*.

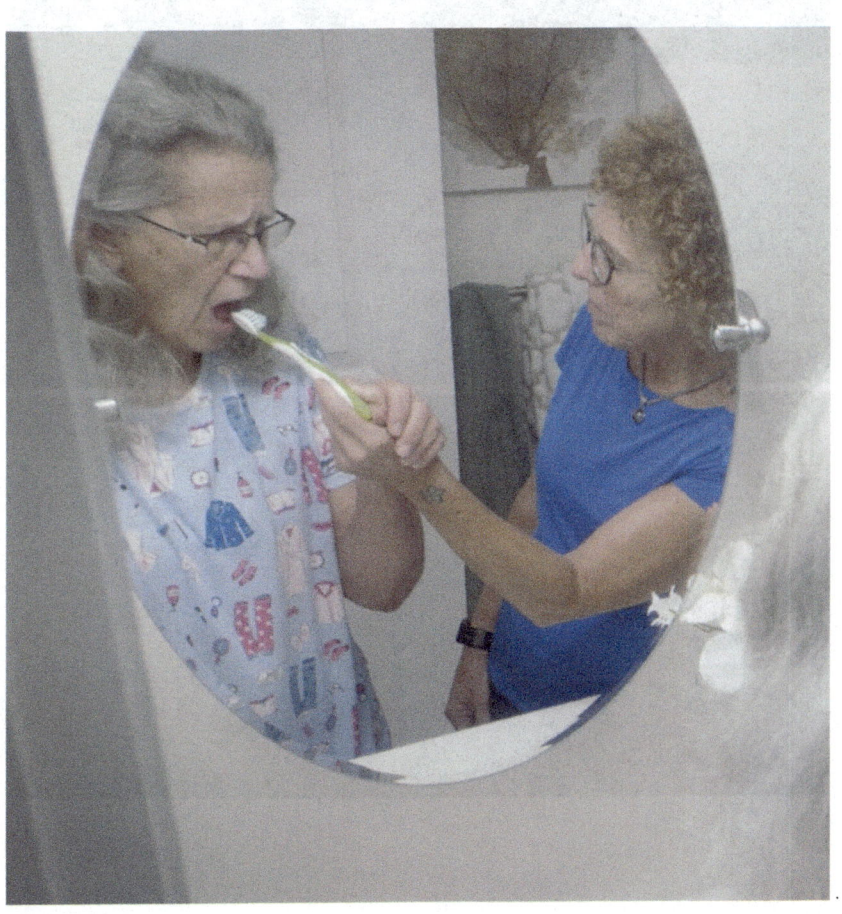

How to Get into the Hand-under-Hand® Position

1. Offer your hand in a typical handshake position. Shake hands, but don't let go.

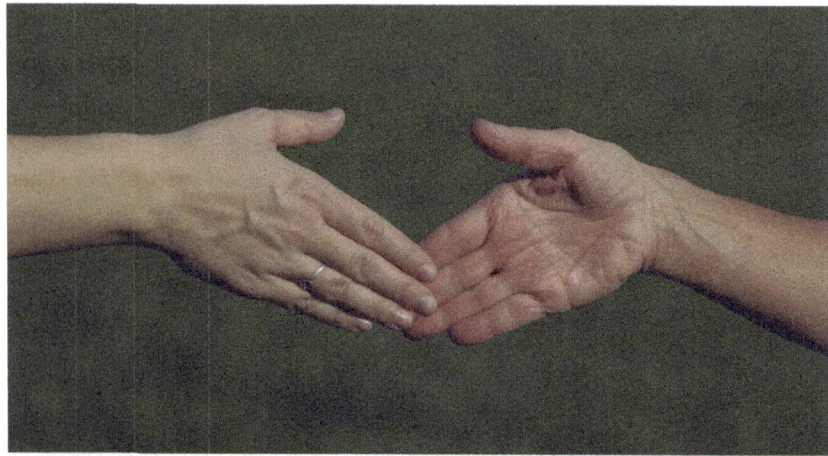

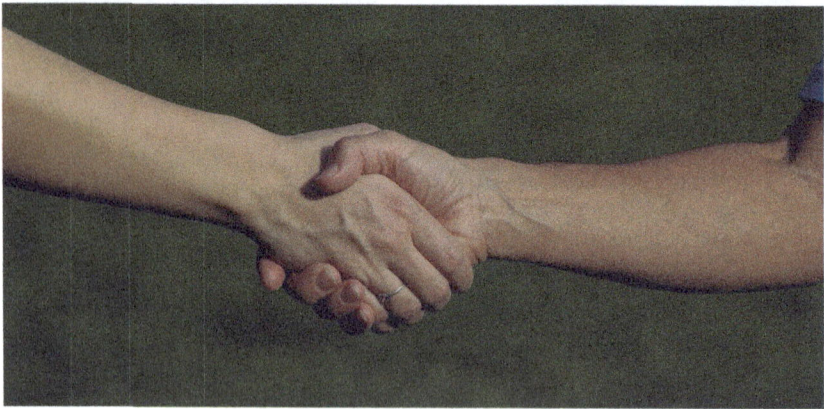

2. Keeping the base of both thumbs in contact, release the fingers and slide the palm of your hand across the other individual's palm, keeping your thumbs pressed together near the base. Wrap your fingers around the base of the other person's thumb. The other individual should also do the same—you can help them gently position their fingers if needed. Because this may take some practice, try this out with someone who can provide you with accurate feedback.

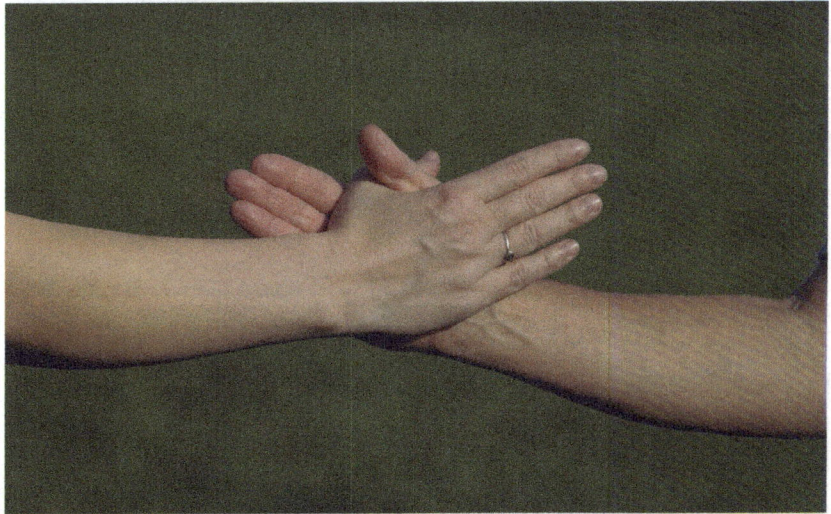

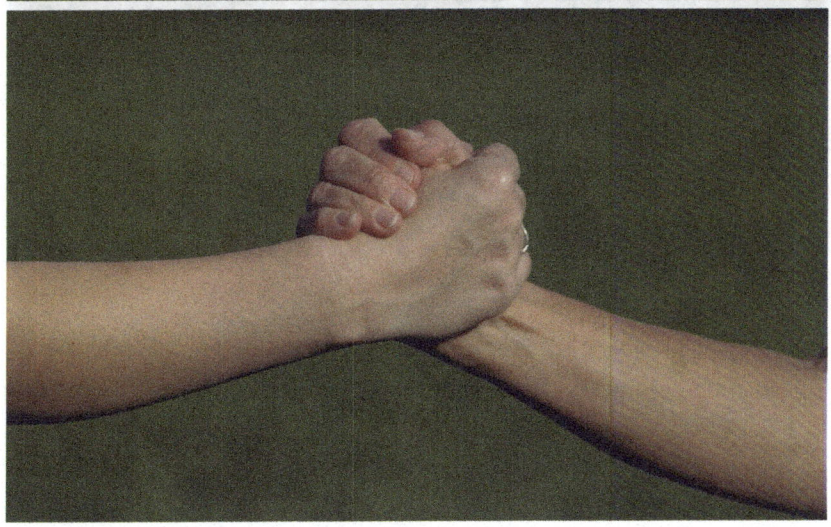

Hand-under-Hand® Support

3. As you are changing your hand positions from handshake to Hand-under-Hand, shift your body to the right side of the individual. Then position your hand so your hand is underneath the other person's hand, supporting it.

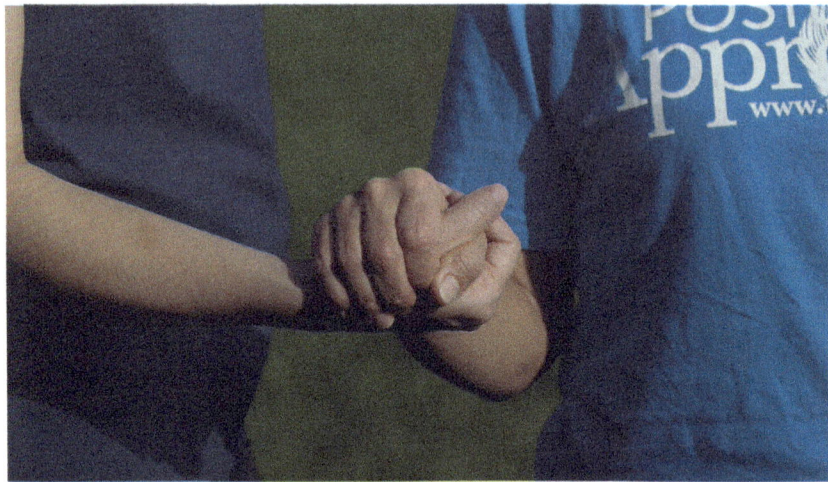

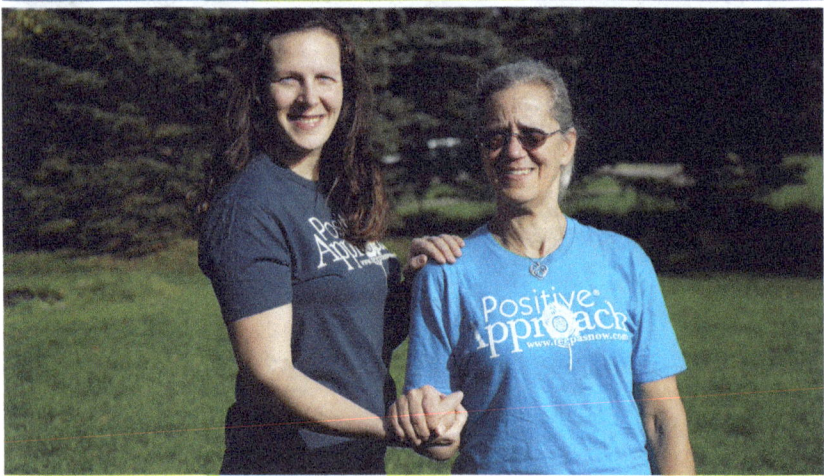

4. Pumps of gentle pressure, with the flats of your pinky and ring fingers into the webspace at the base of their thumb, will help to gain their attention and encourage eye contact. Once again, it is very helpful to practice this skill first with someone who can give you detailed feedback before involving a person living with dementia.

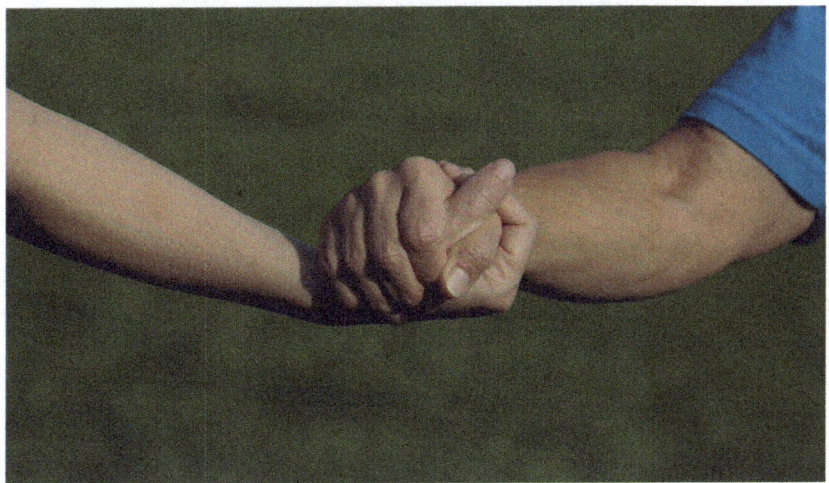

Positive Physical Approach™ (PPA™)

The basis of my overall approach to supporting someone is called a Positive Approach. I want to create a partnership with the person so that we can work together. I don't want to do anything for them or to them without their approval. So, how do I get connected? I refer to this as the Positive Physical Approach.

You'll notice that I use the word *Physical* in the title. Getting connected is more than using words, it's also how I position my body and why. Am I approaching where they can see me or will I surprise them? Am I blocking their field of vision or can they see me but also see past me? Am I leaning in and invading their space, or am I in my space?

While you read this section, see if you can notice the use of Visual-Verbal-Touch (V-V-T) sequencing that has been mentioned throughout this book.

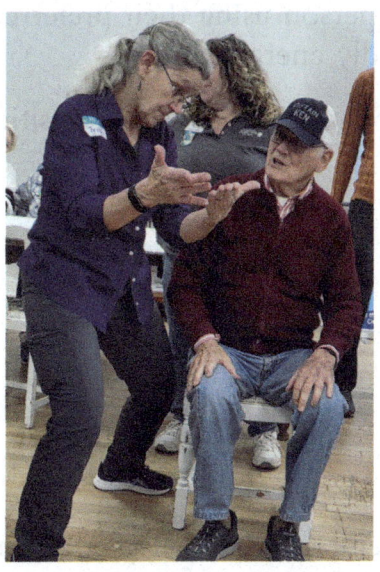

- Try positioning yourself so that you would be in their central field of vision if they were to look up, while being about *six feet away* from them—this is the typical boundary between public and personal space.

- If entering someone's room or personal area, try offering, *Knock, knock!* while knocking on the door, door frame, or table edge, since this is a border of their territory.

- Place your open, *still* hand next to your face and smile when the individual looks at you.

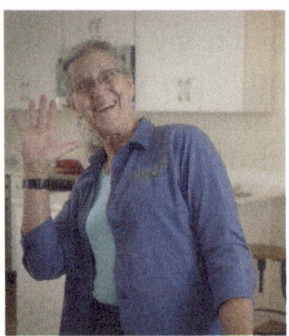

- Greet the person using their preferred name in a clear, friendly, energized voice.

- Offer your hand in a handshake position.

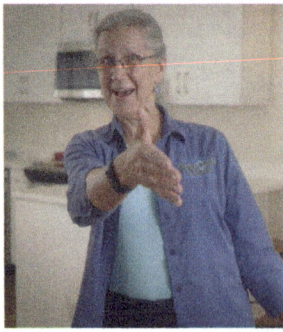

- If they extend their hand, *approach slowly* from the

front, with your hand extended, not talking unless the person has a visual impairment and requires movement/position cues.

- o If they do not extend their hand, stay where you are and consider stabilizing yourself there until you receive permission to move closer.

- Move from the front to their dominant side, getting into a *supportive stance* as you move from the handshake to Hand-under-Hand® position.

  - o For 90 percent of people, the right side is their dominant side.

- Get at or below their eye level by sitting down, kneeling, or squatting; but *don't lean in*.

- If you are not planning on sitting, *lean outward and back* to create a sense of space and equality.

  - o Stand nearly sideways to their body, as if you were on a surfboard, with more of your weight on your back foot.

Did you catch the V-V-T?

- Visual—get in their line of vision but about six feet out.

- Verbal—say their preferred name and then yours.

- Touch—extend your hand for a handshake, but only move forward and touch them if they extend their hand as well. We only touch with permission.

  - o Use a **Positive Personal Connector** (see below) and pause for their response, noting how quickly and accurately the person is able to respond.

  - o Deliver a message using cues and a **Positive Action Starter** (see below) that will help you initiate the next step forward for the interaction or task.

As you look at the steps listed above, you may notice a couple of things:

- You don't necessarily have to do all of these steps in this exact order every time. Consider these steps the ingredients to the recipe and you can decide, with your skill, which steps are needed in this moment without losing the main goal—getting connected and forming a relationship in this moment.

- Positive Physical Approach is more than a way of getting connected. It is also a dynamic assessment that allows you to see what abilities the person has at this moment and also where they may need more support. How quickly are they processing? How are their language comprehension and speech production?

By utilizing the Positive Physical Approach, we are able to join in a partnership for simple connection and task completion. You may be amazed at what a big impact this can have.

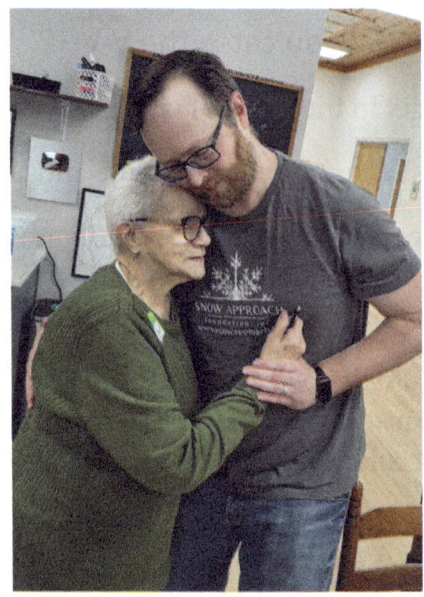

Positive Personal Connectors (PPC)

Now that you have approached using PPA, take time to **Connect:**

- **Greet:** Introduce yourself and use their preferred name.

    "Hi (preferred name), it's (your name)" if known to one another.

    Or

    "I'm (your name), and you are?" if unknown, or uncertain if the person sees you as familiar.

- **Compliment:** Indicate something about them of value.

    "Great color on you!"

    Or

    "You are one of my favorite people!"

    Or

    "You have the best smile."

    Or

    "Wow, you are really good at that!"

- **Share:** First about you, then leave a blank.

    "I'm from (city or state), and you're from?"

    Or

    "I like coffee, and you like . . . ?"

- **Notice:** Point out something in the environment.

  "Boy, that plant has had a lot of love!"

  Or

  "Wow, that is a beautiful _____ (item/object)!"

- **Seek:** Explore a possible unmet like, want, or need.

  "It's a bit chilly in here, a hot drink would be nice. Coffee, or something else?"

  Or

  "You are looking cold . . . ?"

  Offer a visual cue and use a questioning tone of voice.

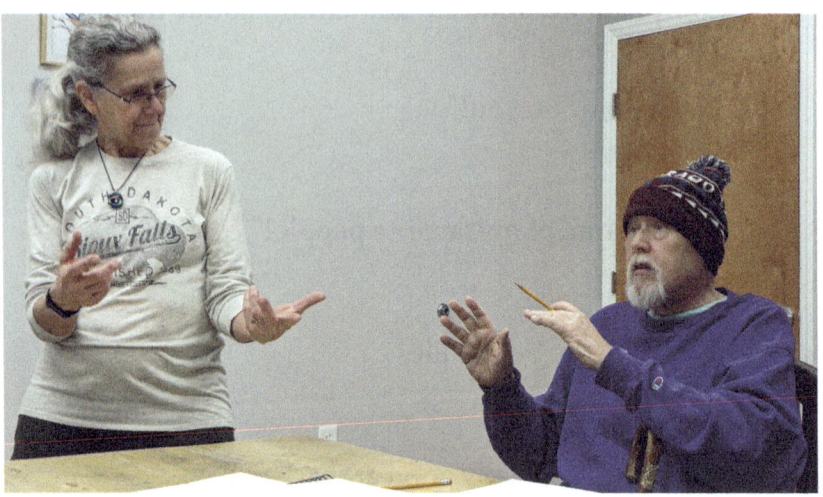

Positive Action Starters (PAS)

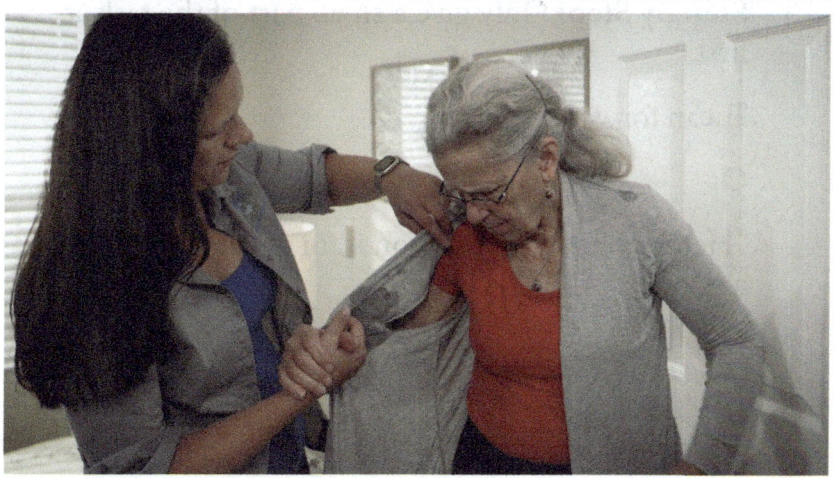

After you have taken a few seconds to connect and you have a better sense of the person's pace, ability to comprehend and respond to language, and the strength of your connection:

- **Help:** Be sure to compliment his or her skill in this area, then ask for help with something.

    "You are so good at _____, I could use your help."

- **Try:** Hold up or point to the item you would like to use, possibly sharing in the dislike of the item or task.

    "I have a favor to ask of you ... give it a try?"

- **Choice:** Try using visual cues to offer two possibilities or one choice with something else as the other option. Could it help to use props versus just words in this situation?

    "This or something else?"

- **Short and Simple:** Give only the first piece of

information, and maybe offer a time frame of one to five minutes.

"It's about time to _____ (first task)."

- **Step by Step:** Only give a small part of the task at first.

"Lean forward."

Or

"Here's your shirt (position it for getting a hand in a sleeve)."

Approaching an Individual Who Is Distressed

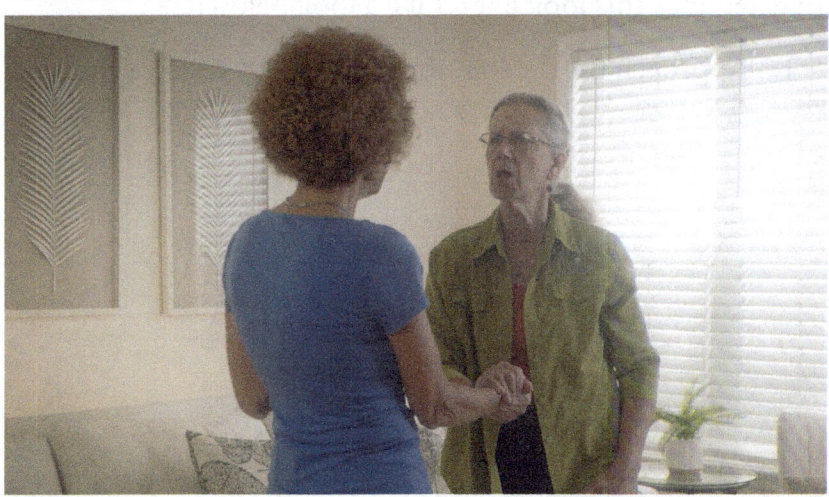

When I introduced the Positive Physical Approach a few pages ago, I was describing a fairly typical situation where the person you are approaching is fine—they aren't in distress. Well, would we do exactly the same thing if the person were in distress? No ... and yes.

What I mean by that is we won't necessarily do all of those steps in that order. However, what we will do is try to connect with the person with a dynamic assessment. Remember what I said about using the ingredients versus following the recipe?

In situations like this, our natural tendency may be to use a calm, soothing voice to get the person to calm down. We may even be tempted to tell them to *calm down*. I have never found this to be helpful, whether I was being told to calm down or trying to help someone else.

While using the philosophy of the Positive Physical Approach, we join the person where they are in this moment. Instead of calm, soothing tones, we try to match their energy level, but just below them. It may seem counterintuitive, like steering into a skid, but this allows the person to realize you understand them, they are being heard, and you are on their side. That makes for a much deeper connection and partnership.

So what does this look like? Take a look below:

1. Approach the person from where they can see you.

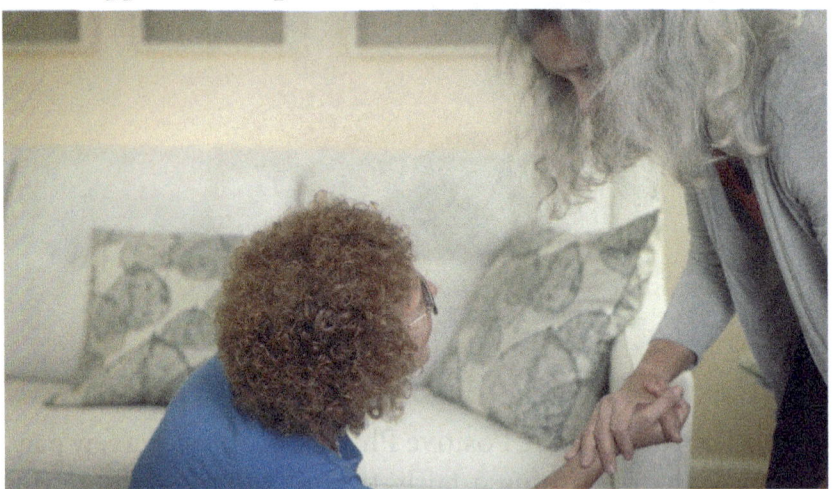

   - Now is not the time to add surprise to what is causing them distress.

2. Stop about six feet out, right on that public/personal space border.

3. Make sure you are in a supportive stance.

   - Stand to their right side, slightly angled so your right shoulder is back and your left foot and arm are more to the front than your right. Shift your weight to your right leg.

4. Reflect the individual's emotion on your face. For example, if they seem sad, display a look of sadness on your face. If they seem angry, show anger.

5. If the person is standing, let the person move toward you, keeping your body turned to the side, even if this means you have to adjust as they move.

    - Glance away if they seem uncertain of you. Try not to stare while you keep their face in your gaze.

6. If the person is seated and you don't get permission to enter personal space, turn sideways and kneel about six feet away from them.

    - Glance away if they seem uncertain of you. Try not to stare while you keep their face in your gaze.

7. If they are able to say what is bothering them, reflect their words back to them in a similar tone of voice.

8. If they don't verbalize what is upsetting them, say, "Sounds like you are (provide an emotion or feeling that seems to be true) . . ."

9. Repeat the person's words. Remember to match their volume, tone, and intensity, but just one level down.

    - If they are saying, "Where's my mom?"
        o You would say, "You're looking for your mom (pause) . . . tell me about your mom . . ." or "You're looking for your mom . . . do you need her for something, or do you just want to be with her?"
    - If the person said, "I want to go home!"
        o You would say, "You really want to go home (pause) . . . tell me about your home . . ." or "You really want to go home . . . do you need to do something there or just be there?"

10. Match the number of words you use with the number of words the person is using. Match their speed and pace, as well.

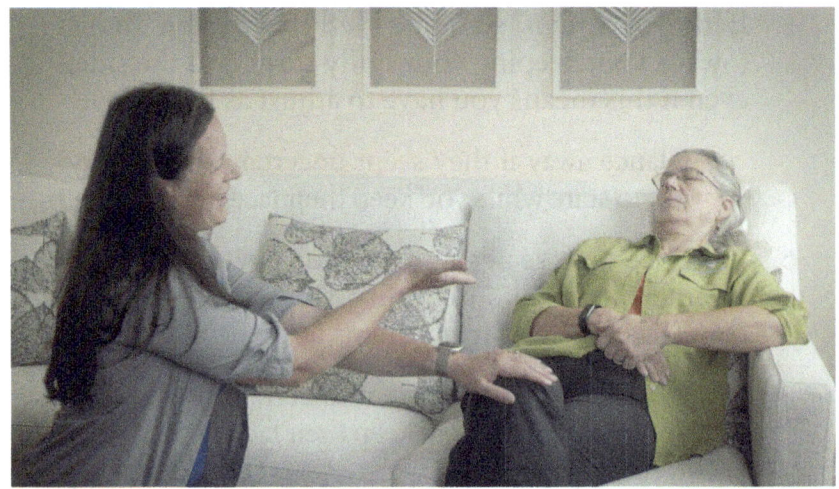

When you form a partnership with a person, even when they are distressed, they will see you as being on their side. This helps create a sense of comfort and will help alleviate the distress.

Situations such as these are often borne out of an unmet need, but you won't be able to fill that need until the level of distress has come down. Once you do help the person come down from that high level of distress, you can become a detective to problem-solve what need is unmet.

On the next pages, you will find some PAC resources to help you with your development of Care Partner Skills.

Our goal is to encourage you to shift from being a caregiver, a giver of care, to a care partner, someone who is partnering with another person or team to provide the best support, guidance, and care possible for all involved.

Other Resources

Teepa Snow's Snow Approach:
Problem Solving Model - Six Pieces of the Puzzle

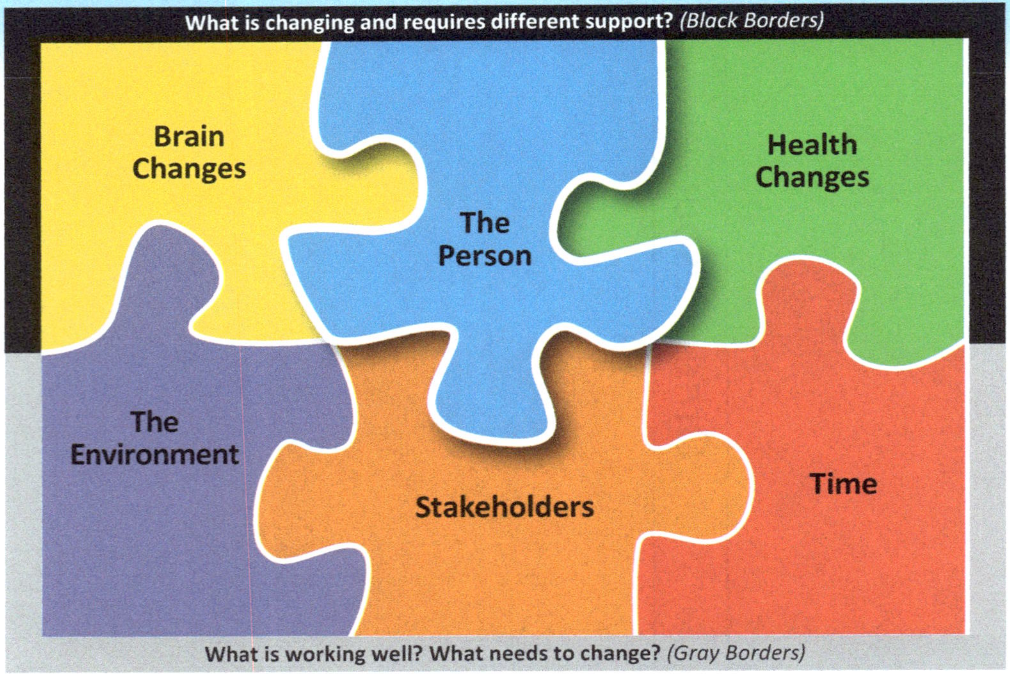

What is changing and requires different support? (Black Borders)

- Health Changes
- The Person
- Brain Changes

What is working well? What needs to change? (Gray Borders)

- Time
- Stakeholders
- The Environment

Life can be challenging for all people and figuring out causes for distress and what helps is critical.

Using these six categories organizes our investigation and keeps us focused and alert.

Supporting each person by using what is possible is the goal.

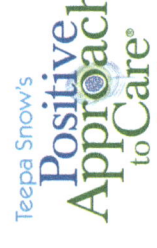

Teepa Snow's Positive Approach to Care®
www.TeepaSnow.com

Copyright © 2006 - 2023 Positive Approach, LLC and Teepa Snow. May not be duplicated or re-used without prior permission. V112023

Dementia Care Partner Guide

What is changing and requires different support? *(Black Borders)*

Brain Changes

Dementia
- Type(s)
- Awareness of changes?

Delirium? Depression or Anxiety? GEMS State(s)
- Changed abilities
- Retained abilities
- Variability
- Onset and duration

The Person

Past and Present
- Life story – history
- Personality traits
- Preferences – likes/dislikes
- Key values
- Joys and traumas
- Roles – watch-talk-do
- Notable positive changes?
- Notable negative changes?

Health Changes

Health Conditions and Physical Fitness
- Intake, throughput, output
- Meds and supplements
- Emotional and psychological condition
- Sensory systems function
- Health beliefs of note
- Recent changes
  - Acute episode of illness
  - New/worsening chronic illness

The Environment

The 5Ps (Place, People, Props, Programming, Possibilities) explore:

The Four Fs
- Friendly
- Familiar
- Functional
- Forgiving

The Four Ss
- Space (intimate, personal, public)
- Sensations (see, hear, feel, smell, taste)
- Surface to Surface Contact (clothing on body, water/air/sun on skin)
- Social (people, activity, role, expectations)

Stakeholders

Care Partner and Others Around
- Agenda(s)
- Awareness, knowledge, skill
- Confidence, competence
- History and background
- Key values
- Personality traits
- Preferences
- Relationship(s)
- Roles - observer, supervisor, carer

Time

Time Awareness
- In the moment, in the present, in the past
- Time of day, week, month, year (season)
- Passage of time (how long since?)

Balance in Four Categories
- Productive: gives value
- Leisure: fun – playful
- Wellness and self care
- Restorative: calm – recharge

Wait Time vs. Engagement in Life Time

What is working well? What needs to change? *(Gray Borders)*

Other Resources 69

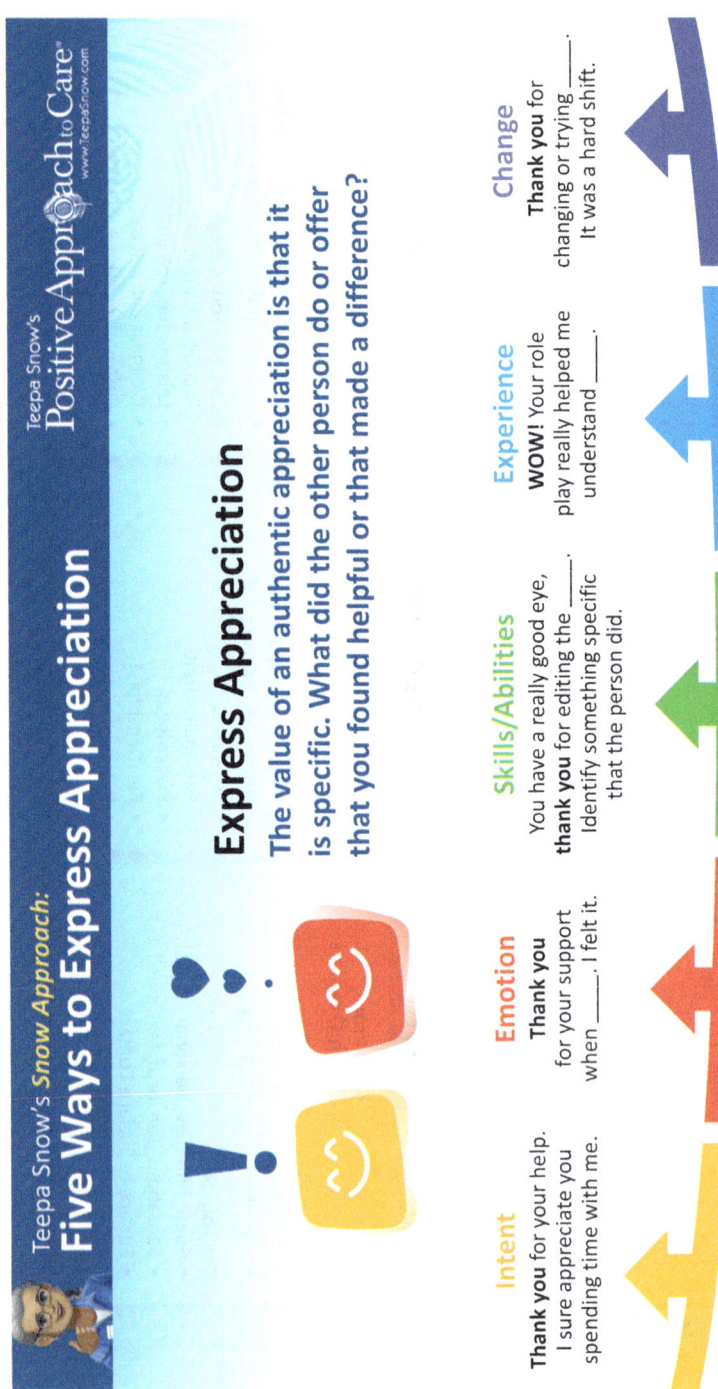

Teepa Snow's *Snow Approach:*
Five Ways to Acknowledge Dissatisfaction

Acknowledge Dissatisfaction

To connect with someone, acknowledge what you are seeing with matching facial expressions and tone. This is a reflection of what you see, not an assumption. Try to say it in a way that invites a response.

It seems like I made you angry = *seek*
I made you angry = *assumption*

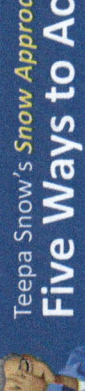

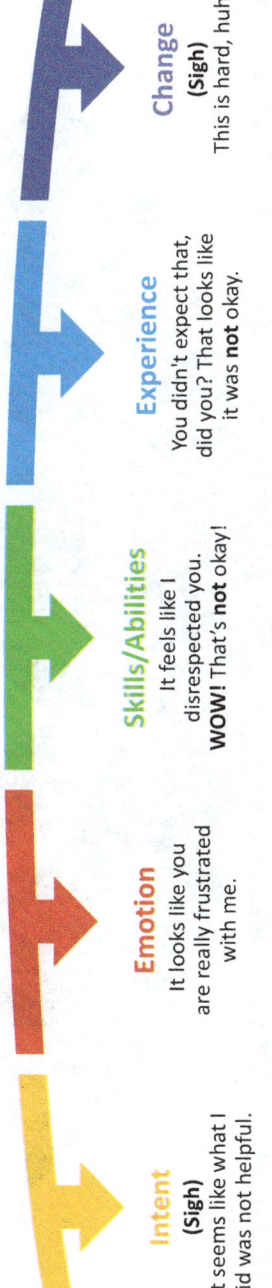

Intent
(Sigh)
It seems like what I did was not helpful.

Emotion
It looks like you are really frustrated with me.

Skills/Abilities
It feels like I disrespected you. WOW! That's **not** okay!

Experience
You didn't expect that, did you? That looks like it was **not** okay.

Change
(Sigh)
This is hard, huh?

Copyright © 2006 - 2023 Positive Approach, LLC and Teepa Snow. May not be duplicated or re-used without prior permission.

V112023

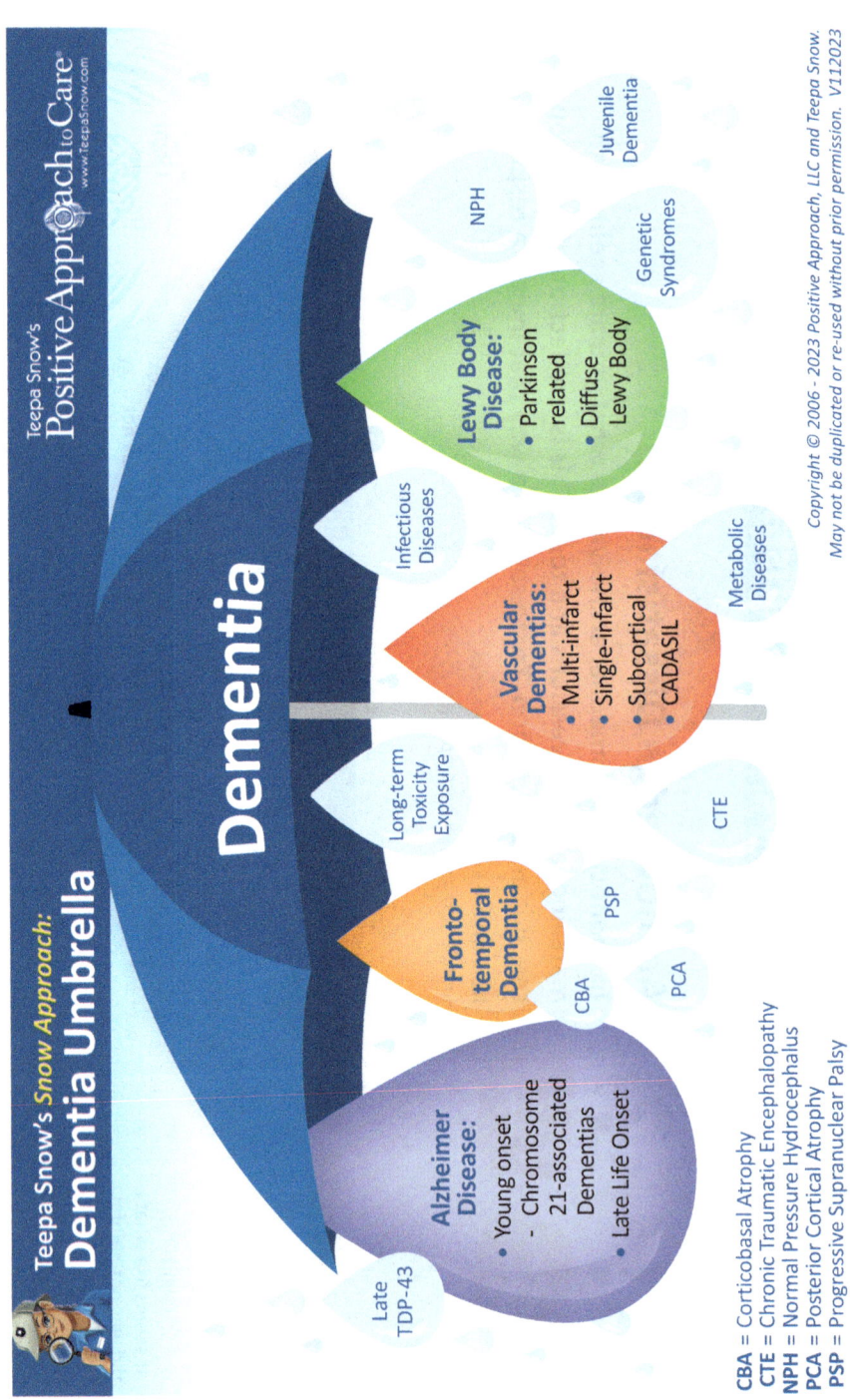

Four Truths of Dementia with Teepa Snow's *Snow Approach*

- Your brain and body will not work the way they used to; abilities are changing, but you will still have abilities.
- It is a new normal; we can't go back to how it was before, but we can adapt.
- It's not going to stay stable and yet, change can be dealt with - with the right support.
- Getting support that works is essential, especially as things continue to change.

Alzheimer

- New details lost first
- Recent memory worse
- Some language problems, misspeaks
- More impulsive or indecisive
- Gets lost – time/place
- Several forms and patterns
- Young onset can vary from late life onset
- Down Syndrome is high risk
- Notice changes over time
- Related to beta-amyloid plaques and tau pathologies

Lewy Body

- Movement problems and falls
- Visual disturbances
- Delusional thinking
- Fine motor problems—hands and swallowing
- Episodes of rigidity and syncope
- Insomnia – sleep disturbances
- Nightmares that seem real
- Fluctuations in abilities
- Drug responses can be extreme and strange
- Related to synuclein protein malformations

Vascular

- Sudden changes in ability – some recovery
- Symptom combinations are highly variable
- Can have bounce back and bad days
- Judgment and behavior not the same
- Spotty losses
- Emotional and energy shifts
- Least predictable
- Caused by problems with blood flow, oxygen, nourishment of brain cells

Frontotemporal

- Many types
- Frontal: impulse and behavior control changes
  - Says unexpected, rude, mean, odd things
  - Apathy – not caring
  - Problems with initiation or sequencing
  - Disinhibited: sex, food, drink, emotions, actions
- Temporal: language change
  - Difficulty with speaking – missing/changing words
  - Rhythm OK, content missing
  - Not getting messages
- Related to tau pathologies

Teepa Snow's
Positive Approach to Care®
www.TeepaSnow.com

Copyright © 2006 - 2023 Positive Approach, LLC and Teepa Snow.
May not be duplicated or re-used without prior permission. V112023

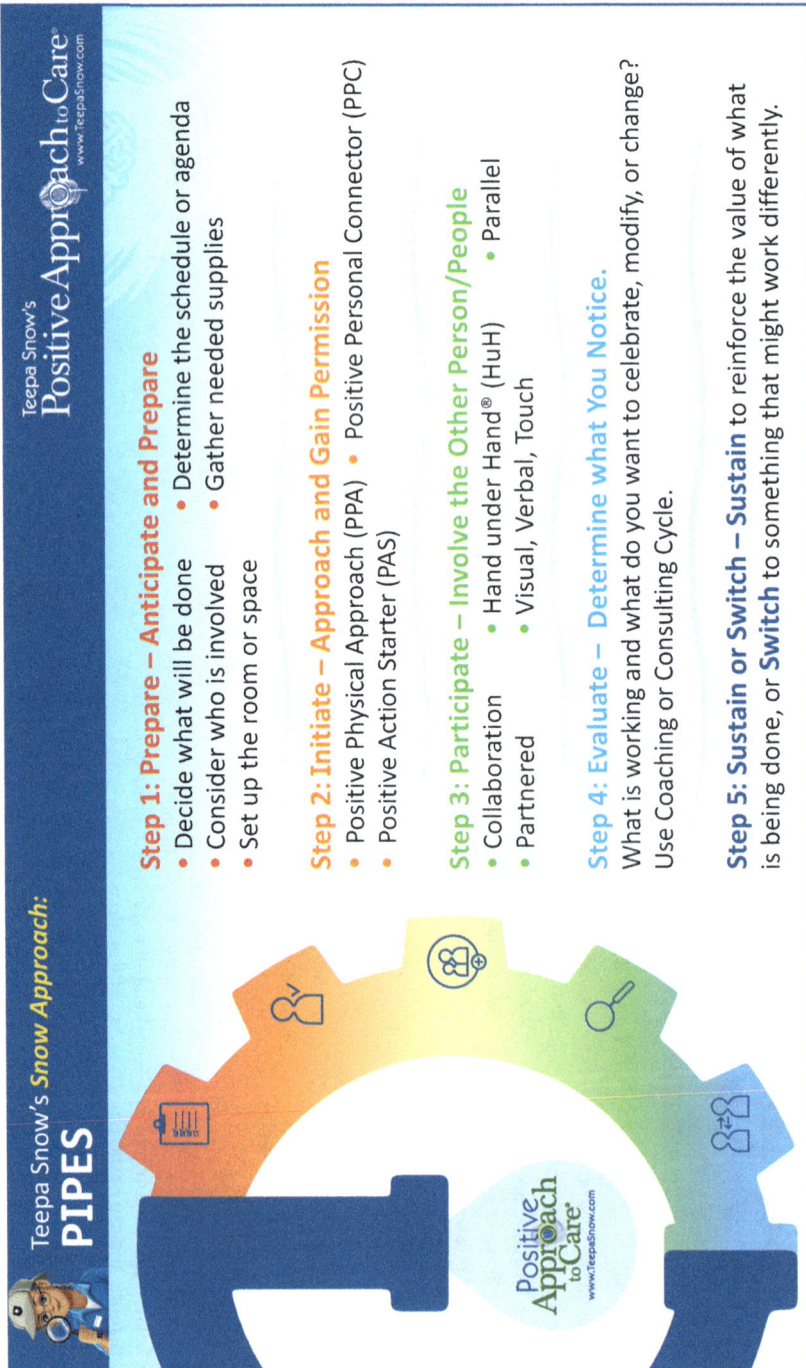

Teepa Snow's *Snow Approach:*
5Ps

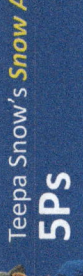

1. Place - What is the physical space involved?
- What in the setting or environment needs to change?
- What is working well?
- What is missing?
- What is not working well?

2. People - Who are the people involved?
- What do we know about them?
- What do they need to be aware of?
- What do they need to know how to do?
- Have they ever seen better interactions or outcomes?

3. Props - What are the physical and visual objects involved?
- What are the objects and items around, and do they meet expectations?
- Are there substitutions or alternatives available to better match interests and abilities?

4. Programming - What is the planned use of time involved?
- How is time being used and how long do people have to wait for support?
- How much time does staff have to offer support for each person?
- What do the rhythms of each day look like for the various people involved?
- Is there balance for all involved of:
  – *Purposeful engagement*   – *Pleasurable enjoyment*
  – *Personal care completion*   – *Rest and restoration periods*

5. Possibilities - What are the possible changes involved?
- What could we try, or what is a new pathway or synaptic pattern we want to attempt?
- How will we know if we are making any meaningful progress?
- Which of the other Ps could/should we vary?

Copyright © 2006 - 2023 Positive Approach, LLC and Teepa Snow. May not be duplicated or re-used without prior permission.

V112023

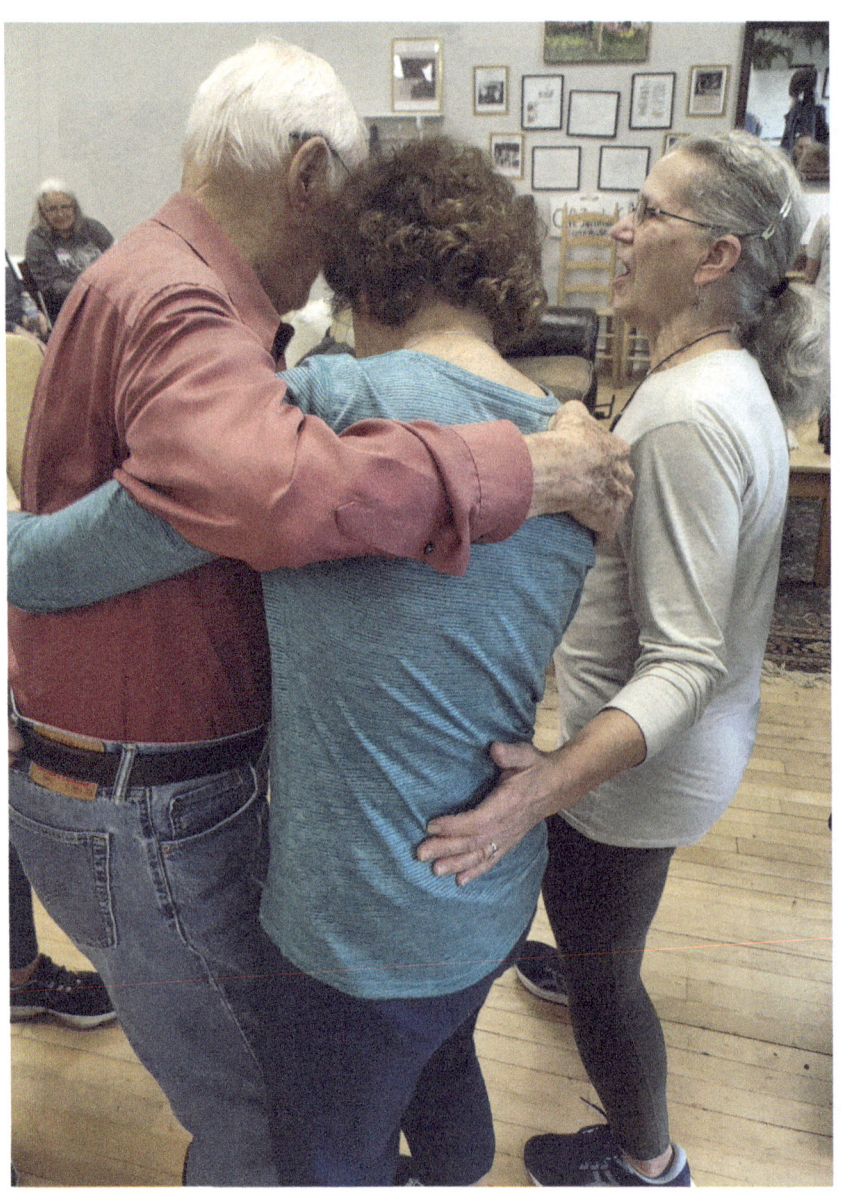

Conclusion

When an individual is living with dementia, it will eventually change almost everything about that person. Dementia is not a memory problem, it is brain change and, ultimately, brain failure. As care partners supporting those living with dementia, we have choices. One choice is that we can try to fight back and battle the disease. The problem with this strategy is that the disease is hidden inside the individual, so it often feels like we are angry and upset with them. Another choice is that we can give up and just let it happen, seeing only what we are losing and the shell that remains.

Or we can choose to commit ourselves to learning how to let go of what is fading, but celebrating and using what remains at any point in time. We can decide to become care partners on this journey, not caregivers or those who step away because she doesn't know who I am anymore. Each person must make the choice for themselves. You cannot make it for another.

Being a care partner is hard. There may be times when it hurts and times when you need a break or a partner yourself. You will make mistakes. You are human and you cannot get it right the first time, every time. When you are trying to think for another individual, it doesn't always work out the way one or both of us would like it to. The goal in dementia is to plan for the worst probabilities, but celebrate the best moments! The one constant in this ever-changing condition can be your commitment to travel with someone as they make the journey. To do this, you must plan to change as the condition changes the person's ability to process incoming information and data, to respond or react to what happens and how it happens, and even to thrive as you learn to live in this world.

The following points are important to keep in mind:

- Many times, when we are surprised or frustrated by something, it is not the person, it is the disease.
- We can use what we see, hear, feel, and experience with the person to guide our behavior.
- Interacting will require us to work hard and not just do what comes naturally in many situations.
- We must learn to respond, rather than react, as there may be moments when the only thing we can do is stop and step away to gather ourselves. Remember, first, do no harm.
- Old patterns, habits, or relationship triggers can cause our brains to shift brain states quickly and intensely.
- To be successful care partners, we will need to let go of what was, what should be, how the person should be, and how we should be; and simply live in the moment we are given.

I hope this guidebook helps each of you on your unique path through the journey of dementia.

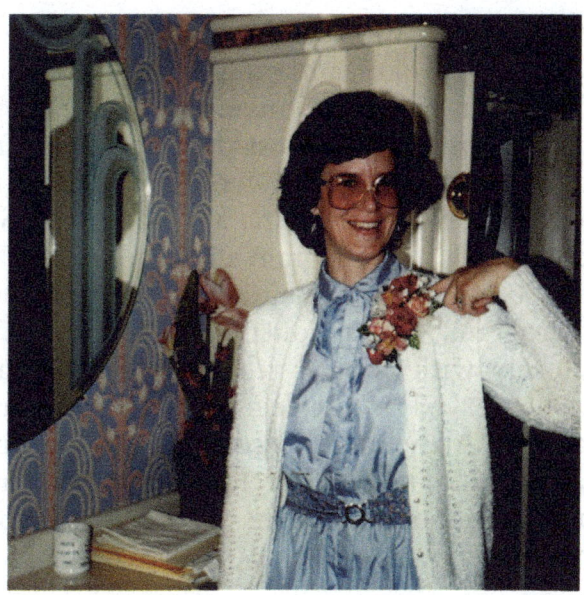

About Teepa

Teepa Snow is an Occupational Therapist with over forty years of clinical practice and teaching experience in a wide variety of settings. She developed her knowledge and skills through her rich and diverse life and work experiences. Teepa began her journey as a care partner as a young girl when her grandfather came to live with her family. At the time, her grandfather was described as becoming senile. Teepa found she was much better at helping her grandfather get through the day than her mother, who became easily frustrated with repeated questions and unrealistic expectations. That early experience with her grandfather helped to shape her career and direction. She later provided care and support to other family members who developed forms of dementia.

Teepa has worked in hospitals, rehabilitation centers, retirement communities, nursing homes, home care, hospice, and community settings. She has extensive experience in neurological care settings, working with people who have had head injuries, strokes, and other central nervous system failures. Teepa has taught at universities and colleges from an associate degree to the post-doctoral level, including appointments at the Duke University School of Nursing, the University of North Carolina at Chapel Hill School of Medicine, and was the program director for the Durham Technical Community College's Occupational Therapy Assistant Program. Throughout her career, Teepa has also worked closely with clinical researchers in geriatrics. In addition, she served as the lead trainer and educational director for the Alzheimer's Association in Eastern North Carolina, where she helped develop training programs and videos for national organizations that support those living with dementia.

In 2007, Teepa founded her company, Positive Approach to Care® (PAC). PAC provides online and in-person education and products to support those living with brain change, with the mission of creating a more inclusive global community. In 2022, Teepa cofounded Snow Approach with her daughter, Amanda. Snow Approach Foundation, Inc., is a nonprofit organization based in Hillsborough, North Carolina. When she is not busy with her organizations, Teepa presents extraordinary expertise and humor to audiences throughout the world and spends time with friends who are living with various brain abilities. She also enjoys taking risks that challenge those around her.

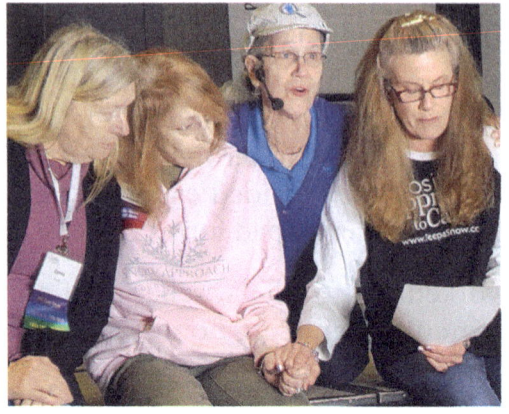

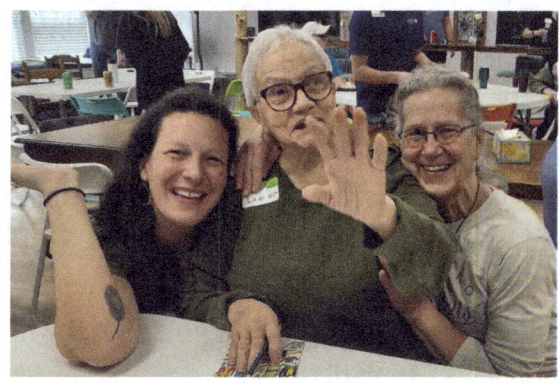

Being a care partner is hard. There may be times when it hurts and times when you need a break or a partner yourself. You will make mistakes. You are human and you cannot get it right the first time, every time. When you are trying to think for another individual, it doesn't always work out the way one or both of us would like it to. The goal in dementia is to plan for the worst probabilities, but celebrate the best moments! The one constant in this ever-changing condition can be your commitment to travel with someone as they make the journey. To do this, you must plan to change as the condition changes the person's ability to process incoming information and data, to respond or react to what happens and how it happens, and even to thrive as you learn to live in this world.

The following points are important to keep in mind:

- Many times, when we are surprised or frustrated by something, it is not the person, it is the disease.

- We can use what we see, hear, feel, and experience with the person to guide our behavior.

- Interacting will require us to work hard and not just do what comes naturally in many situations.

- We must learn to respond, rather than react, as there may be moments when the only thing we can do is stop and step away to gather ourselves. Remember, first, do no harm.

- Old patterns, habits, or relationship triggers can cause our brains to shift brain states quickly and intensely.

- To be successful care partners, we will need to let go of what was, what should be, how the person should be, and how we should be; and simply live in the moment we are given.

I hope this guidebook helps each of you on your unique path through the journey of dementia.

Thanks for choosing to
make a difference!

Leepa

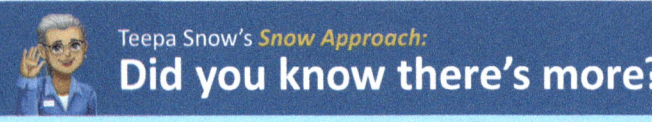

Teepa Snow's *Snow Approach:*
Did you know there's more?

Teepa Snow's Positive Approach to Care (PAC) offers a variety of care partner, professional, and organizational training tools and services.

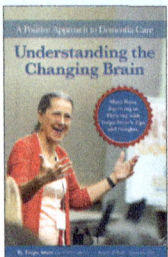

Understanding the Changing Brain

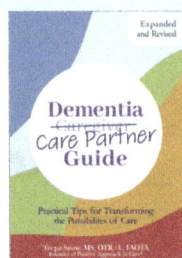

Dementia Care Partner Guide Expanded and Revised

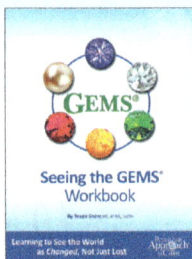

Seeing the GEMS Workbook

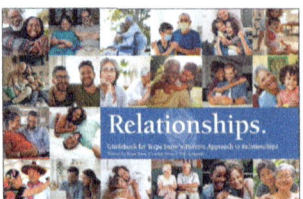

Relationships. Guidebook for Teepa Snow's Positive Approach to All Relationships

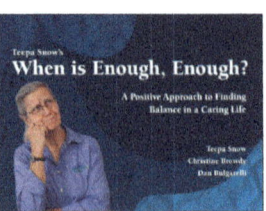

When is Enough, Enough? A Positive Approach to Finding Balance in a Caring Life

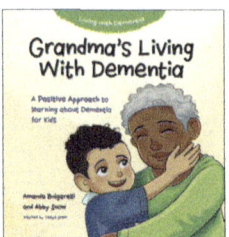

Grandma's Living with Dementia

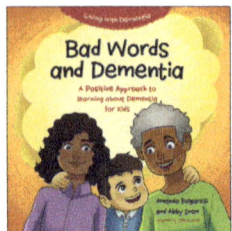

Bad Words and Dementia

Discounted Bulk Products

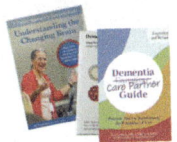
Books

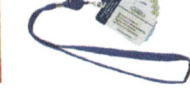
Skills Cards

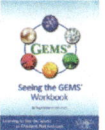
GEMS Workbook

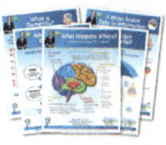
Mini Poster Set

Certification Courses
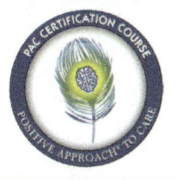

Organizational Trainings
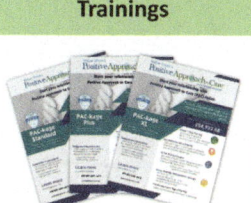

Videos Streaming or DVD
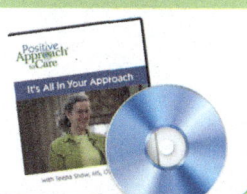

Live Workshops and Skill Building
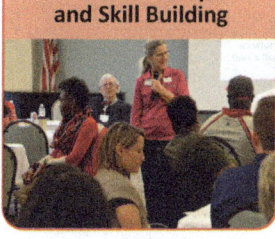

One-on-One Consultations
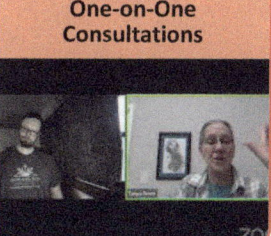

Care Partner Support Series
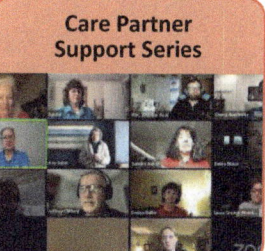

For more details and to learn about the best fit for you:

Visit our
Website
www.TeepaSnow.com

Visit our
Store
shop.TeepaSnow.com

Teepa Snow's
Positive Approach to Care
www.TeepaSnow.com

info@TeepaSnow.com
877-877-1671
Follow us on social media!

Copyright © 2006 - 2024 Positive Approach, LLC and Teepa Snow. May not be duplicated or re-used without prior permission. V042024

Made in the USA
Monee, IL
30 August 2025

24653617R00059